Your Ch

Your Child With Asthma

Some Advice for Parents and Others

SIMON GODFREY, M.D., Ph.D., M.R.C.P.
Consultant Paediatrician

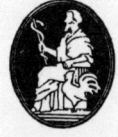

HEINEMANN HEALTH BOOKS
London

First published 1975

© Simon Godfrey 1975

ISBN 0 433 12300 1

Text set in 11/12pt Photon Imprint, printed by photolithography,
and bound in Great Britain at The Pitman Press, Bath

This book is for Joanne, Joseph, Alisa and Charlotte
who haven't wheezed
and for Andrew, Wendy, Kevin and Charles
who have

CONTENTS

	Preface	vii
	Acknowledgments	viii
Chapter 1	The Nature of Asthma	1
2	The Causes of Asthma	9
3	The Patterns of Asthma in Children	22
4	Investigating the Asthmatic Child	32
5	The Treatment of the Asthmatic Child	49
6	Who Should Treat the Asthmatic Child—and Where?	69
7	Some Important Rules for Parents	82
	Index	87

PREFACE

This book is really intended for the parents of children with asthma, to give a straightforward account of what we know about the course of the disease and its treatment. It is hoped that the book will also be of interest to others who have contact with asthmatic children, particularly schoolteachers and people involved in activities such as youth clubs, scouting, etc. Although an attempt has been made to write the book in terms that the ordinary person can understand, it may also be of some interest to medical students and even doctors who will often have to face the parents of an asthmatic child.

I have written this book to try to provide some explanations to the very common problems which parents raise when I see them in the children's asthma clinic. One of the chief objectives of the book is to give a reasonable account of childhood asthma and its treatment, and to destroy some of the myths and old wives' tales which surround the subject. The first part of the book describes the way in which the lungs work and the way they are affected by asthma, and then goes on to discuss the various causes of the disease. Next follows a section describing the usual course of asthma in children and the way that it may be investigated in the hospital clinic. The last part of the book concerns the various kinds of treatment that are available for the asthmatic child and also discusses who should be responsible for the treatment and where it should be carried out. However, this book is not intended as a "do-it-yourself" book on asthma for parents, who must of course consult their usual medical adviser about the treatment of their child. Its real purpose is to explain why doctors give the advice that they do.

For readers who wish to have a simple but reasonably full account of childhood asthma the best course is to read the book

Preface

through from beginning to end. Some people may not be very interested in the explanations of the normal working of the lungs and its disturbance in disease, which is contained in Chapter 1, and they might like to start later in the book or to use the index to find the topics of particular interest to them. At the end of the book, in Chapter 7, I have summarized the important messages for parents in the form of a set of nine simple rules. I believe that the lives of asthmatic children and their parents, not to mention their doctors, would be made much easier if these rules were kept in mind. In some ways the last rule is the most important of all, and this states that "Your child probably has 9 out of 10 chances or better of completely losing his asthma by the time he reaches his teens."

ACKNOWLEDGMENTS

This book is the result of experience I have gained over a number of years in treating children with asthma both at the Brompton Hospital and at the Hammersmith Hospital in London. During this time I have benefited from the discussions and advice I have received from many colleagues, both medical and non-medical, who are too numerous to mention individually but to whom I am indebted all the same. Much of my research into the problems of asthmatic children has been made possible by support from the Medical Research Council and the Asthma Research Council, to whom I am greatly indebted. I should also like to thank the parents of my patients who have helped me to clarify my thoughts on this subject and particularly to those parents who have read the proof of this book and offered me their advice. The index for the book was prepared very efficiently by my wife, Dr. Carole Godfrey, and the manuscript was typed by Mrs Valerie Chalk.

CHAPTER I

The Nature of Asthma

Introduction

The parents of the asthmatic child usually have a very clear idea of what is meant by asthma because they see that their child suffers from repeated bouts of difficult and wheezy breathing. It seems strange, therefore, that doctors often disagree when they try to define asthma in medical terms and that different names such as bronchitis, wheezy bronchitis, spastic bronchitis, or asthmatic bronchitis may be used by different doctors when describing the same asthmatic child. Some of this confusion between asthma and bronchitis is due to the fact that asthma in adults is often complicated by chronic bronchitis with excessive production of sputum, or with other lung diseases. Fortunately, these problems are much less common in children and it is easier to reach a definite diagnosis. Another reason for confusion is that a true attack of bronchitis, which means inflammation of the bronchial tubes, is often caused by a virus infection and this virus can also cause an attack of wheezing in the asthmatic. Parents know from experience that a cold may "go to the chest" and cause wheezing in their asthmatic child.

It is necessary to know something about the structure and function of the lungs in order to understand the basic disturbances which occur in asthma. The roles of infection, allergy, and emotional and physical factors which can provoke attacks of asthma can then be seen in their true perspective.

The Structure and Function of the Lungs

All animals produce energy by burning up food with oxygen and this process releases carbon dioxide as a waste product. It is the function of the lungs to extract oxygen from the air to get rid of the carbon dioxide. In air-breathing animals the lungs are constructed like bellows so that the air goes in and out through a series of tubes arranged like the stem and branches of a tree—the bronchial tree as it is often called.

The breathing apparatus of man consists of the upper air passages (nose and mouth), the larynx (voice box) and trachea (wind pipe), the smaller air passages (bronchi) and finally the tiny air sacs at the end of the finest bronchi in which gas exchange occurs (alveoli). These structures are shown diagrammatically in Figure 1. We normally breathe through our noses and small babies are often unable to breathe through their mouths at all. Any form of obstruction in the nose will therefore affect the breathing, especially in babies, and this can sometimes be confused with asthma. The situation is complicated by the fact that asthmatic children often develop obstruction of their noses as well.

The chief structure of concern in asthma are the air passages below the larynx (usually called "airways" in medical terms) because it is in these lower airways that the blockage occurs in asthma. The wind pipe branches into two main bronchial tubes, one going to each lung. Each of these tubes branches again into two smaller tubes and so on, for a total of about 15 to 20 generations of branching. This means that there are something like 14 million of the smallest bronchial tubes in both lungs together. This number of tubes is present at birth,

The Nature of Asthma

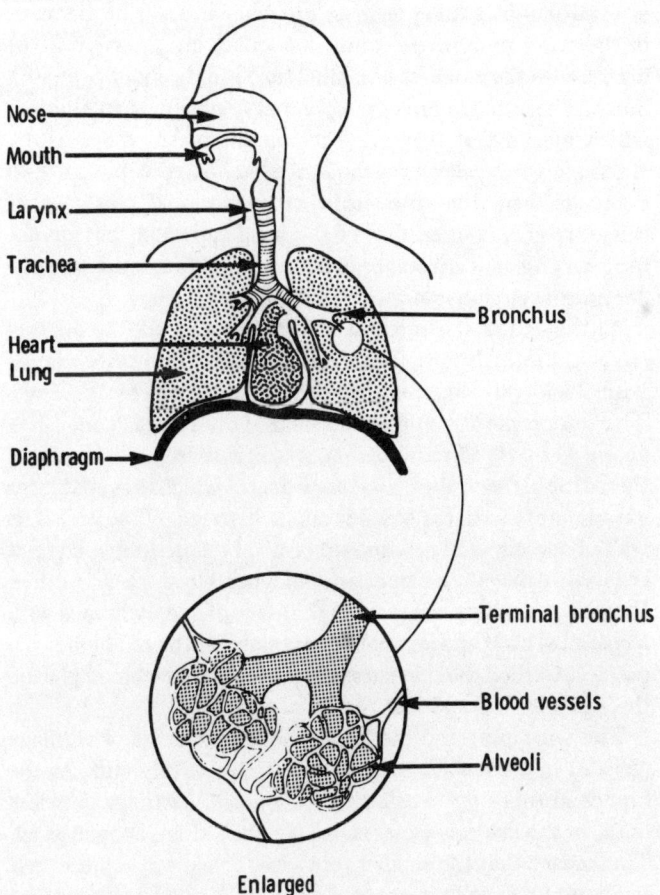

Enlarged

Fig. 1. Diagram to illustrate important parts of the airway and lungs. The inset shows an imaginary magnification of one of the endings of the bronchial tree to show the air sacs (alveoli) with their walls surrounded by blood-vessels.

so that the lungs grow by adding on air sacks and increasing in size, but not by adding on more bronchial tubes. The diameter of the wind pipe in the adult is about $\frac{3}{4}$ in. (2 cm.) but the diameter of the smallest bronchial tube is only about $\frac{1}{50}$ in. (0·5 mm.). These tubes are correspondingly narrower in children which means that they can become obstructed more easily. Although the smaller bronchial tubes are narrow, there are so many of them that their total cross-sectional area is considerably greater than that of the wind pipe and they do not form a significant resistance to air flowing through the lung under normal circumstances.

At the end of the smallest bronchial tubes are the air sacs (alveoli) in which the gas in the lungs comes into close contact with the blood being pumped through the lungs by the heart. There are some 300 million alveoli in the adult, each one being about $\frac{1}{100}$ in. (0·25 mm.) across. Because there are so many of these tiny air sacs, their total surface area which is available for gas exchange with the blood is about 90 sq. yd. (75 sq. m.). The wall of the air sac is composed of a very thin double layer of cells with the air on one side and the blood on the other. Oxygen passes outwards through this wall and combines with a chemical called haemoglobin contained in the red blood corpuscles. Carbon dioxide passes inwards from the blood plasma through the wall and into the air sac.

The wind pipe and the larger tubes have rings of cartilage (gristle) in their walls so that they are relatively stiff. As the bronchial tubes get smaller the amount of cartilage gets less until, in the last few generations of tubes, there is none at all. This means that the smaller tubes can be squashed flat rather easily and this may occur if a great deal of effort is used to breathe out in an attack of asthma. Almost all the bronchial tubes also have muscles in their walls which can contract and reduce their width. These muscles are not under voluntary control, but like the muscles of the gut, they are controlled un-

The Nature of Asthma

consciously and normally help to stiffen the walls of the bronchial tubes. In the asthmatic subject these muscles may become over-active and go into spasm (bronchospasm), making it more difficult for gas to flow through the lung. The bronchial tubes are lined by cells which keep them lubricated and remove any unwanted particles by gently sweeping them up and out through the larynx. Excess production of lubricant is coughed out as sputum. In asthma, the lining cells may become swollen and produce excessive secretions which also contribute to obstruction of the airways. In very severe attacks the sections may form thick plugs which block off quite large tubes.

In order to take in oxygen and remove carbon dioxide, the lungs have to be moved like bellows and this is done by the diaphragm and the muscles of the chest wall and abdomen. If the bronchial tubes are unduly narrowed by an attack of asthma, their resistance to gas flow is increased and extra muscles are used to help the patient breathe, especially the large neck muscles. Because the smaller airways tend to get squashed during expiration, not all the normal amount of air can escape when the patient breathes out and this means that he must breathe with a larger volume of air in his chest. Normally, the lungs are so efficient at taking up oxygen that all the haemoglobin in the red blood corpuscles is converted into its oxygen-carrying form which gives the blood a bright red colour. In an attack of asthma, the mechanical disturbances to gas flow in the lungs may mean that gas and blood do not meet in the correct proportions in the air sacs. The result is that some of the haemoglobin is not fully converted and the blood has a bluer colour. If this is very marked, the patient's lips and tongue will also take on a bluish tinge (cyanosis), but this is quite rare in asthma. It is also rare for an asthmatic patient to experience any problem in getting rid of carbon dioxide because this gas can be blown out of the lungs very easily.

The Effect of Asthma on the Structure and Function of the Lungs

The characteristic feature of asthma is temporary narrowing of the bronchial tubes which makes it harder for the patient to move air in and out of his lungs. Even in health there is a certain resistance to flow of air through the tubes (airways resistance), but during an attack of asthma this resistance is considerably increased. The narrowing of the bronchial tubes can result from the exaggeration of the normal contraction of the muscles in the walls of the bronchi, from swelling of the cells lining the tubes, and from excessive secretion of fluid into the tubes (Fig. 2). In childhood asthma it is usually the muscular contraction (bronchoconstriction) which is most important, but the other factors also contribute. When the attack is over, either spontaneously or in response to treatment, the

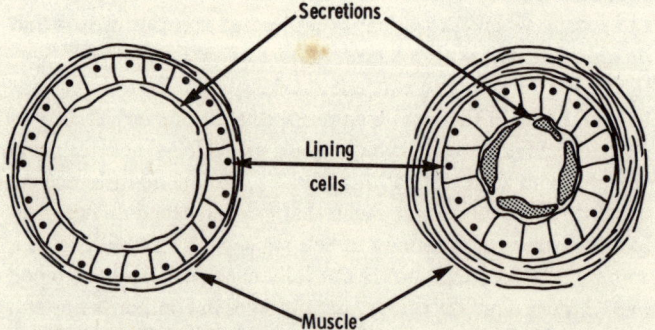

Fig. 2. Diagram to illustrate the changes that occur in the bronchial tubes during an attack of asthma. All three processes of contraction of the muscle, swelling of the lining cells, and increased secretions contribute towards narrowing of the air passage.

The Nature of Asthma

bronchial muscles relax and the tubes open up (bronchodilation).

The resistance of the bronchial tubes varies during the breathing cycle because they are pulled more open as the lungs enlarge during inspiration. This means that the asthmatic finds it easier to breathe in than to breathe out. Because of the tendency to trap air in the lungs the patient must breathe in to a larger lung volume, and big muscles of the neck and shoulders are used to help the diaphragm. The extra large forces needed to overcome the airways resistance during an attack are also reflected in the sucking in of the spaces between the lower ribs and above to collar bones which can often be seen in a child. Clearly, all the extra work used to move air in and out of the lungs can be very tiring in a prolonged and severe attack of asthma. The disturbance of movement of air together with this fatigue may contribute to the abnormally low level of oxygen and occasionally high level of carbon dioxide in the patient's blood.

The most important feature of asthma is the great variability in the level of airways obstruction, and this is seen very clearly in children. Other lung diseases, such as chronic bronchitis or emphysema, also cause increases in airways resistance but they never show the variation seen in asthma and they produce a fixed type of increased resistance due to permanent damage to the walls of the bronchial tubes. In contrast, children with asthma rarely have any permanent damage and the narrowing of their bronchial tubes is due to alterations in the state of the bronchial muscles and lining cells which reverses easily. Even during an attack of asthma the level of obstruction may vary from hour to hour or from morning to evening. As will be seen later, this variability of childhood asthma can make it quite difficult for the doctor to assess the severity of the child's condition.

The characteristic ability to vary the degree of airways

resistance in an asthmatic can be demonstrated by the inhalation of one of the drugs which can relax the bronchial muscles. This usually produces a complete or partial relief of the obstruction and easing of the breathing, which does not occur to anything like the same extent in a patient with chronic bronchitis. The bronchial tubes of the asthmatic are also sensitive to factors which can increase the level of resistance, such as inhaling pollen if he is allergic to it. In fact, it is this lability ("twitchiness") of the bronchial tubes which really distinguishes the asthmatic from the normal person and from patients with other diseases. Bronchial lability can also be demonstrated by asking the child to run about for a few minutes. This often results in a brief attack of asthma which begins when he stops exercising. Exercise-induced asthma can be produced even between regular asthma attacks when the child is otherwise well, and is sometimes quite troublesome during sports activities.

The breathlessness and discomfort of the child during an attack of asthma can now be seen to result from the simple interference with lung function which occurs. Airways obstruction distorts the normal pattern of breathing and requires harder work while at the same time causing disturbances of oxygenation of the blood. The essential point to grasp, however, is that it should be possible to completely reverse the abnormalities in the asthmatic child.

CHAPTER 2

The Causes of Asthma

Asthma is a very common disease which is estimated to affect about 1 in 10 of all children at some time. It has been recognized and written about since ancient times and the effects it produces on the body are well known. Despite all this information, it is very rarely that a doctor can answer truthfully when asked by parents about the cause of their child's asthma. And because of this uncertainty, a whole host of theories have been developed about the cause of asthma, which are often no more than old wives' tales. Some physicians believe that asthma is all due to allergies, others believe that it is all due to infections or physical factors such as the climate, while still others believe it is all due to emotion or "nerves". When faced with this confusion within the medical profession, it is hardly to be wondered that parents are even more confused themselves. Fortunately, most physicians will treat the child with the best available methods, whatever they may consider to be the cause of the asthma, so that the doctor who thinks it is due to allergy will also treat any emotional disturbances, and the doctor who thinks it is due to "nerves" will also use drugs which relax the bronchial muscles. Because parents, and sometimes physicians, may become unduly worried about what label they should use to describe the cause of the child's asthma, this chapter sets out to explain some of what is known about the role of various factors.

Your Child With Asthma

The Role of Allergy

Allergy is a term which has come to be used very loosely by the general public, especially in North America, and has therefore lost some of its meaning. The patient who breaks out in a rash every time he takes penicillin is undoubtedly allergic to the drug, but the patient who feels unwell after eating eggs but can eat cakes and other food prepared from egg without trouble is probably not allergic to them.

In the medical sense, allergy is used to describe a common abnormality of one of the most important defence mechanisms of the body—the immunological defence system. This system enables the body to detect and destroy bacteria or viruses and to remove any of its own cells which have developed abnormally. The immunological defence system consists of certain specialized cells in the blood and other tissues, and a series of complex chemicals in the blood called immunoglobulins. A good example of the beneficial working of the immunological defence system is the protection given to children by immunizing them against diptheria when they are young. An extract obtained from diphtheria germs (not the actual germs themselves) is injected and the body builds up a defence system of cells and immunoglobulins. If the child is attacked by a real diphtheria germ later on in life, the defence is already there and the invading germ is rapidly destroyed.

The processes which occur in an allergic patient are similar to those occurring in the normal immunological defence system, but differ in the ease with which they are brought on and the sites at which the reactions occur. All the people living in one area are exposed to the same amount of pollen, but the normal subjects do not develop hay fever or asthma, even though they recognize pollen as foreign protein. The allergic patient recognizes foreign proteins very easily and is particularly good at making a special type of immunoglobulin

The Causes of Asthma

called IgE (pronounced IGE). This IgE attaches itself to cells called mast cells and then lies in wait, so to speak, in the walls of the bronchial tubes, nose or eyelids. When the pollen comes along, it is recognized by IgE and this reaction triggers off the mast cells which liberate various chemicals causing other cells to swell, bronchial muscles to constrict and blood vessels to dilate. If these reactions occur chiefly in the nose and eyes, the patient has hay fever, and if they occur chiefly in the lungs he has asthma. Of course, the reaction can occur in both sites at the same time. It must not be thought that all allergic reactions are of the type described because there are other mechanisms, too complex to consider here, by which they can occur. However, the simple allergic process described is a good example of the way allergy works.

One interesting property of the IgE immunoglobulin is that it attaches itself to mast cells in the skin. This means that it can be shown up by the reaction which occurs in the skin when a small amount of a substance to which the patient is allergic is injected. This is the basis of the skin tests which are used to check for allergies. When the test substance, called an allergen, is pricked into the skin it reacts with the IgE on the mast cells and liberates chemical agents which cause a small, itching bump to appear and then slowly subside. The majority of asthmatic adults and about 90 per cent of asthmatic children show this type of positive skin test to one or more allergens, of which the commonest are pollens, house dust, animal products and foods.

The fact that the great majority of asthmatic subjects can be shown to have allergy on skin testing has naturally led many people to believe that the asthma is caused by allergy and that the removal of the allergen should lead to a cure. Unfortunately, the position is not quite as simple as this. There are a number of asthmatics, even children in whom we cannot demonstrate any allergies, and, conversely, positive skin tests are found in about 20 per cent of normal subjects who do not have asthma. Moreover, it is very common to find evidence of allergy to a particular substance by skin testing even though the patient has never noticed any asthma coming on after contact with the offending allergen. For example, a positive skin reaction to cat or dog fur may be found in an asthmatic child whose attacks began before the pet was bought, was unchanged after its arrival and continued after it was removed.

Despite the rather negative evidence given above, there can be little doubt that allergy plays a major role in the lives of most asthmatic children. In some cases it seems to be almost entirely responsible for the attacks, as for example in pollen asthma which only occurs in the spring and early summer, or in the occasional patient who always gets an attack as soon as he comes into contact with a particular animal, food or medicine. These purely allergic forms of asthma do occur and the diagnosis is almost always made by the alert parents who notice the unfailing attack of asthma which follows contact with the allergen. A much more common allergic factor in asthma is house dust, or rather the tiny mite which is found in house dust in almost every home in all parts of the world. This mite is particularly plentiful in and around bedding since it lives off the scales shed from skin. Control of dust in the bedroom seems to help many asthmatic children and positive skin tests to the mite occur in almost all young asthmatics.

The true place of allergy in the causation of childhood asthma needs careful consideration. In many cases it is just one of a number of factors which can spark off an attack or prolong the period of wheezing. Unless there is a clear-cut association between the allergen and the asthma attacks, then the finding of positive skin tests is probably not important. On the other hand, when there is a close link between the allergen and the asthma, especially if the skin test is very positive and if inhaling or eating the substance can be shown to provoke an attack, then the allergy may be very important indeed.

The Role of Infection

The place of infections in causing asthma is still not entirely clear, but it is now known that virus infections are particularly important in childhood asthma. Part of the difficulty is that it may be quite difficult to actually find the offending germ, especially if it is a tiny virus, without highly specialised laboratory investigations. Most attacks of childhood asthma are treated by family doctors who do not usually have these laboratory facilities, but some very important investigations have been done by family doctors who have detected viruses in a high proportion of asthma attacks in children. These studies have shown that the same virus affecting a family will cause a simple cold in normal children but wheezing in asthmatic children. Another problem about the role of infection is that the symptoms of an attack of asthma may resemble those associated with infection itself. For example, the asthmatic child often has a persistent and very annoying cough which is usually found with bronchitis or other chest infections in adults. In the asthmatic child, this cough occurs without any evidence of infection and is probably caused by irritation of the narrow bronchial tubes. To complicate matters, patients with asthma provoked by an allergy often have watering eyes and a running nose before or during their asthma attack. These symptoms are of course quite typical of the common cold but it does not mean that the asthmatic is infected with the common cold virus just because he has similar complaints.

Just as some attacks of asthma are quite clearly provoked by virus infections, some attacks are accompanied by infections with bacteria, which are larger types of germ. The important difference between these organisms is that viruses are not killed by antibiotics like penicillin, but bacteria can be destroyed by suitable drugs. This is the reason why many doctors treat asthmatic children with antibiotics—just in case a bacterial infection is at the root of the trouble. In hospital it is usually possible to do tests to find out if a bacterial or viral infection is involved before giving an antibiotic. It must be emphasized, however, that the majority of asthma attacks in children are not improved by antibiotics because they are not caused by bacterial infection and the improvement seen during treatment would have occurred on its own.

It is often believed that infections of the tonsils or adenoids are an important cause of asthma in children. The tonsils and adenoids are special areas around the back of the throat and nose which have the function of helping to pick up and destroy any invading germs. Because of this they often become inflamed, especially in children where contact with germs causing this type of infection is rather frequent. If the tonsils or adenoids are removed, the defence takes place deeper inside the body. There is no evidence that taking out tonsils or adenoids reduces the incidence of asthma in the child, and these important tissues should not be removed unless there are very special reasons such as deafness or severe ear infections. Similar arguments are often put forward to suggest that infection of the sinuses around the nose contribute to the child's asthma. It should be remembered that obstruction of the nose in an asthmatic may well be due to an allergy and not to infection at all. However, if there is real evidence of sinus infection and not just simply a blocked nose this may be important.

The Role of Emotional Factors

"Asthma is due to nerves, isn't it doctor?" This is one of the commonest questions based on popular folk lore that is asked of the doctor treating asthma. Some doctors believe that the

The Causes of Asthma

answer is "Yes", and even more believe that the answer is "No". In fact both these extreme views are wrong and the correct answer is, "Asthma attacks are sometimes provoked or made worse by nerves." It is very important to remember that asthma can be a very frightening experience for the child who feels he cannot breathe and for the parents who have to watch him struggling for breath. If such attacks are allowed to recur without adequate treatment, the child and his parents can easily become extremely anxious and if the child senses his parents' anxiety his own nervousness may get worse. Once in a panic, the child often makes very forceful attempts to breathe, and, as explained in the first chapter, all he succeeds in doing is to compress his bronchial tubes even further. It is easy to see how this sequence of events could be misinterpreted to suggested that the child's asthma is due to "nerves".

The situation may progress even further with the development of the so-called "typical" asthmatic mother and child. What is usually meant by this is that the child can apparently manipulate the other members of his family and his mother fusses and is over-protective. Some asthmatic children seem to be able to turn on an attack when they do not get their own way or when they are faced with an awkward situation. Other children may be unduly shy and sensitive or aggressive and jealous. It must be realized, however, that all these personality types occur in non-asthmatic children and there is absolutely no evidence to suggest that the personality causes the asthma. In fact, it is interesting to see how many so-called "nervous" asthmatic children improve in terms of their personality and behaviour once effective treatment is started to control their wheezing. Children with other types of chronic illness, such as diabetes or rheumatism, also have emotional problems and their mothers often become over-protective. It is more likely that these are the normal reactions of a family to ill health in a child, especially if the disease is frightening.

Your Child With Asthma

What has been said above does not mean that emotional factors have nothing to do with the child's asthma. There is no doubt that in some children frustrations or anxieties within the family may provoke or exacerbate their attacks. It is well known that a child may become worse with the arrival of a resented younger brother or sister, or if there is strife between the parents. Some children have very severe asthma at home which vanishes as if by magic when they go away to boarding school, only to return during the holidays at home. Likewise, a severely asthmatic child may improve dramatically within hours of admission to hospital, having received no treatment at all. Parents are often upset by this type of reaction, believing that it means that they are responsible for their child's asthma. It cannot be emphasized too strongly that there is no evidence to support this idea and that we cannot yet explain the apparently beneficial effect of leaving home.

It is quite simple to demonstrate that emotional factors do affect asthmatic children, just as they can affect children with other diseases. This is particularly clear when new treatments are being tried out and the patient is given either the active drug or a dummy preparation in order to see if the new treatment really works. In almost every case there is definite improvement in the asthma when the dummy treatment is given, though of course it is not so marked as the improvement when an effective drug is given. The improvement with the dummy occurs because the child and his parents believe that it will help and just as emotional factors can make the asthma worse, so they can also make it better.

Some asthmatic children may become very disturbed indeed, but this is quite unusual and the incidence of true mental illness is no higher amongst asthmatics than amongst other children. Some psychologists have proposed very elaborate theories to explain the development of asthma; for example, it has been thought to represent suppressed crying at the thought

The Causes of Asthma

of separation from the mother. Again it must be stressed that there is no evidence to support such ideas at the present time, and the search for such hypothetical causes may well do a disservice to the asthmatic child. On the other hand, many asthmatic children have emotional problems which deserve and require as much attention as their physical problems. Provided both aspects are considered with common sense, then the correct answer to the question, "Is it all due to nerves?" will usually be, "No, but they may be helping to make it worse."

The Role of Environmental and Physical Factors

It is commonly believed that climate has a lot to do with asthma and parents with badly affected children often ask whether they should move or send their child to live in a supposedly better environment. Many children are in fact sent away from home to live in such places as Switzerland and Arizona, and many of these children are much better than when they lived at home. However, it was noted above that improvement often occurs in asthmatic children when they leave home or are admitted to hospital, even in their own city. Some of the benefit attributed to climatic change is really due to removal from home. In addition, children often go to live in the different climate when they are about 8 or 9 years old, at the height of their disease, and return home when they are in their teens when the disease normally tends to become less troublesome. This spontaneous improvement is often mistaken for the effects of a "good" climate.

If we look around the world it is obvious that there is no such thing as a really good climate in which children do not get asthma, and the disease is found in children from cool, damp areas like Britain, from warm, dry areas like Australia, from low-lying areas like Holland, and from mountainous areas like

Colorado. On the other hand, practical experience has shown that some children do improve when they move to another climate and some are made better or worse by changes in weather. It is quite possible that some children have bronchial tubes which are very sensitive to the temperature of the air and their asthma may well be affected by changes, but it must be stressed that the weather itself does not cause the asthma—it merely acts as a triggering mechanism. It can be seen that the question of moving to a different climate is very complicated and many different factors could be involved in any improvement (or lack of it) which occurs.

One of the most striking factors which causes asthmatic children to wheeze is physical exercise. Most asthmatics find that certain types of exercise, especially running, will bring on a brief attack even if they are otherwise well, and it will certainly make them worse during an ordinary attack. This so-called "exercise-induced asthma" may be such a prominent feature of the child's disease that he is quite unable to play normal games with his friends or take part in sports at school. Such children are often thought to be very delicate and many asthmatic children are not allowed to take exercise in case it brings on an attack. In fact, if the exercise-induced asthma is prevented by treating the child with an appropriate drug, then he can do just as well as a normal child in sports. It is also important to realize that different types of exercise have different effects in the individual, and the child may be able to play soccer or swim but not do athletics. As with the other factors considered, exercise does not cause the asthma but acts as a trigger mechanism to bring out the wheezing. Preventing the child from taking exercise will not cure him of his asthma and making him exercise will not make the basic disease worse, although it can bring on a quite severe attack in some cases. In general, the child should not be made to persist with the type of exercise that is known to make him wheeze unless he is given effective preventive

The Causes of Asthma

treatment, but exercise which does not upset him should be allowed.

Sometimes excitement, laughing, crying or deep breathing can bring on an attack of asthma. This is sometimes mistakenly taken as evidence for an emotional cause of the disease, but in fact these activities are acting as triggers in very much the same way as exercise. Whether due to exercise or any of these other activities, the attack can be reproduced in the laboratory by having the child run, laugh, overbreathe, etc., without the involvement of any allergic, emotional or infective factors.

The Role of Inheritance and Sex

Without doubt, the most striking thing about children with asthma is the predominance of boys and the presence of disease in other members of the child's family. This has led us to believe that inheritance is a very important factor in determining whether or not a child will become asthmatic. The sex difference is really very striking in children, with the boys outnumbering girls by at least 2 to 1. It is interesting that the difference disappears in young adults, and in older patients women may outnumber men. It is very common to find that one or both parents and brothers or sisters have asthma, hay fever or allergic skin disease, either as children or adults. About one quarter of the close relatives of an asthmatic child will have active or previous asthma and another quarter will have hay fever or skin allergy. About two out of every three relatives will have positive skin tests for allergy and about one in three will have an abnormal response to exercise tests. All these figures are very much higher than we should find amongst the relatives of a normal child, and they emphasise the very strong hereditary factor in asthma. It should not be imagined that the pattern of inheritance of asthma is quite simple and that a child will not have asthma unless his parents have the disease. There

Your Child With Asthma

are a proportion of children in whom no family history of asthma exists in the immediate relatives, but it will often be found that grandparents, uncles, aunts or cousins have had asthma or one of the related conditions mentioned. There is also no doubt that asthma occurs in some children in whom there is no trace of the disease in the family.

One very difficult obstacle in a simple inherited theory of asthma is that identical twins do not always both have the disease. With non-identical twins one would only expect the same frequency of asthma between them as between non-twin

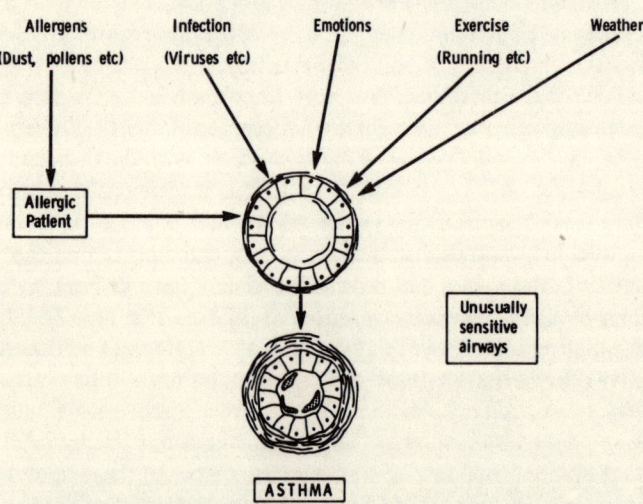

Fig. 3. Diagram to illustrate possible ways in which an attack of asthma can be provoked. The patient has unusually sensitive airways, probably as an inherited condition, and all the various provoking factors can act either alone or in combination on these airways to cause them to narrow.

The Causes of Asthma

brothers and sisters, but identical twins have exactly the same inheritance from their parents and therefore should have identical asthma if it were inherited simply. There have been a number of reports in the medical literature of identical twins, one of whom has asthma and the other not, or in whom the severity of asthma is different in the twins. However, in almost all cases there is some trace of inherited abnormality as shown by tests for allergy or bronchial lability. This shows that environment as well as inheritance is important in determining the occurrence of asthma.

It seems likely that the inherited factor is very important in most children but it only serves to prepare the ground, so to speak, so that the child can develop asthma if the disease is started up by some other event (Fig. 3). There is some evidence to suggest that virus infections in childhood may start up the asthmatic tendency, but there is no reason to believe that it could not also be started up by allergy, other infections or emotional factors. This may be the reason why so much confusion has existed about the cause of asthma.

To summarize the position about the causes of asthma, it may be said that any theory which suggests that one or other factor is the sole cause of asthma in children should be viewed with great reservation. There is no doubt that allergy, infection, physical factors and emotion all play a part in lighting up or modifying the child's condition, and it is highly likely that their contributions vary from child to child. There is a strong inherited factor in asthma but it probably takes some outside event before the inherited tendency results in the disease. There is precious little evidence to suggest that climate or environment can cause asthma apart from its influence on the other factors already considered.

CHAPTER 3

The Patterns of Asthma in Children

Each individual asthmatic child has his own particular pattern of disease and must be treated in the light of his own experiences. However, certain features of the disease are so common that it is possible to describe typical examples of the course it may run. Even before starting this description, it must be stressed that there is no guarantee that any given child will stick to a particular form of the disease and he may well change from one to another. It is unwise to predict anything about the likely course of events in a child from what has gone before, even though we may have a good idea what the "average" asthmatic may do.

The course of the disease can best be followed by considering children at three very characteristic stages of their lives, that is as babies and toddlers, between about 4 and 10 years of age, and from 10 until they have passed through puberty.

Wheezy Babies and Toddlers

There is absolutely no doubt that the majority of asthmatic children begin to have symptoms when they are quite young babies, even in the first few months of their life. In fact, 80 per cent of children with asthma attending a hospital asthma clinic begin to wheeze before the age of 4 years. This does not mean that every baby who wheezes has asthma since a very large

The Patterns of Asthma in Children

number of babies have one or two chest illnesses with wheezing and never have any more trouble for the rest of their lives. This problem of the wheezy baby has caused a great deal of misunderstanding in medical circles and in the general public, and the situation is still not completely clear. Parents, and even their medical advisers, often fear that a baby who wheezes or has difficulty with breathing will become an asthmatic, but only about 1 in 10 babies who wheeze in the first year of life will grow up to be asthmatic. The older the wheezy baby, the more likely he is to have asthma later, and about 4 out of 10 wheezy toddlers over 3 years old will continue to have attacks. From this it can be seen that wheezing in infancy is far more common than asthma in childhood.

What then is the matter with this relatively large number of wheezy babies? Many of them have infections of their bronchial tubes with viruses, particularly a virus called the respiratory syncytical virus. Because they are so small and their bronchial tubes are so narrow, the swelling caused by the infection can apparently cause some obstruction to air flow through the tubes and so the baby wheezes and blows up his chest just like an asthmatic. The same type of infection in older children or adults will only cause a cough because their bronchial tubes are that much wider. Sometimes, babies have an even more severe variety of this type of illness and are said to have bronchiolitis, which means that we think the infection is in the really fine bronchial tubes. Occasionally the child may have pneumonia which can only be diagnosed for certain with a chest X-ray. One of the distressing and troublesome features of the wheezy baby is that the illness may recur a number of times and does not seem to respond well to treatment. An attack of asthma, even if very severe, can usually be controlled with drugs of one type or another as we shall see later on. Wheezy babies respond poorly or not at all to these types of drugs and this is one of the important pieces of evidence that

Your Child With Asthma

they are not always just infant asthmatics. If the wheezy baby is given good nursing care and attention is paid to his oxygen, food and fluid needs, he usually recovers very well in about a week. The trouble may recur once or twice over the next few weeks or months, but eventually the attacks stop.

Since the majority of asthmatic children start to have symptoms as babies, it would be handy if we could pick them out from all the other wheezy infants who are not going to be asthmatics. Unfortunately, it is rarely possible to do this with certainty before the age of 3 or 4 years, because there is nothing which definitely marks them out. There are certain suggestive features of the disease which are seen in most asthmatic children. For example, it is very common to find that one or more close relatives of a child with asthma has the disease themselves, or has one of the related conditions such as hay fever, nasal obstruction, or skin disease. This family association is also more common in the families of wheezy babies and if very marked would tend to suggest the possibility of asthma. Likewise, a very rapid improvement with the type of drug which is successful in treating asthma, or even a very rapid improvement without treatment, might suggest early asthma, since the ordinary type of wheezy baby responds poorly.

One of the very characteristic features of childhood asthma is the association it has with infantile eczema. This is a skin condition which causes a rough, scaly, itching rash in certain areas, especially over the backs of the knees, the front of the elbows and the cheeks. It can also be much more widespread and varies greatly in severity. Infantile eczema often begins within the first few days of life and disappears after a variable period of time in the great majority of infants. In some cases it may persist as a skin disease without any other problems, but in an important group of children it is associated with asthma. In fact as many as 6 out of 10 asthmatic children have infantile eczema at some time. It may be present from infancy and often clears up before the asthma stops, or it may persist. The actual severity of the eczema does not seem to be directly related to the severity of the asthma, but there is a very curious dependence of one condition on the other in many children. These patients seem to alternate between having troublesome asthma and troublesome eczema, so that when one condition improves the other gets worse, and vice versa.

As time goes by, it generally becomes easier to pick out the truly asthmatic toddler because of the features of his disease which we have discussed above. It is still very unwise of any doctor to give a child under the age of about 4 years the label of asthma, with all it implies for the next few years, because many of them just don't turn out the way one expects.

Asthma in Younger Children

Although most asthmatic children actually begin to have symptoms of their disease when they are quite small, they generally do not have any real problem from repeated attacks until they are a bit older. This can be seen from the fact that about 90 per cent of children attending a hospital asthma clinic are over the age of 5 years and only about 10 per cent need to attend regularly before this age. The pattern of asthma seen by the doctor will depend very much on where he practices. The hospital-based children's doctor will tend to see more severely affected patients than the family doctor. There are three general patterns seen in children, the mild infrequent attacks, the severe infrequent attacks, and the frequent attacks or continuous asthma. In addition, there is the condition known as "status asthmaticus" which really means a severe and prolonged attack which requires rather active treatment and which can occur in any asthmatic irrespective of the general pattern of his disease.

Probably the commonest of all types of asthma in children

consists of mild attacks which occur at rather long intervals, that is about 2 or 3 times a year, over a number of years. The attacks last a few hours to a day or so and in between attacks the child is completely well. Each attack settles down on its own or with the help of relatively mild drugs and many of these children never need hospital treatment. Although there are no definite rules, it seems that this very mild type of asthma tends to keep to the same pattern from the early attacks until it eventually burns itself out. A more troublesome form of childhood asthma also consists of infrequent attacks separated by long intervals of good health, but the attacks themselves are more severe. The child may begin to wheeze, often after developing a cold with a running nose, and rapidly becomes more distressed. He finds it difficult to breathe, especially to breathe out, and he prefers to sit up so that he can use his powerful neck muscles to help him move the air in and out of his chest. These attacks often seem to get worse overnight and may continue on for a few days or even a week. They usually require fairly active treatment and may even need to be treated with powerful drugs such as steroids (see Chapter 5), but after recovering from the attack the child is quite well until the next time.

Both of these intermittent types of asthma may occur more commonly at one time of year than another. Usually the attacks are more frequent in winter since they are often provoked by virus infections which are themselves commoner in winter. Some children are worse in the spring or summer and we always suspect that allergy to pollens may be important in these cases. It is not often realised that attacks at this age are more common at night than in the daytime and the child may go to bed well, only to wake in the small hours with his attack. Young children have a great deal of cough with their attacks, and in fact they may not complain of wheeze at all, just of cough. The child who has attacks of night time cough, or who regularly coughs after exercise, should always be considered as

The Patterns of Asthma in Children

a possible asthmatic, though admittedly the majority of such children will turn out to be perfectly well.

The most common type of childhood asthma seen in hospital clinics is the continuous variety, because this presents most problems for treatment. The usual story is that the child began to have trouble with his breathing as an infant and later on he started to have definite asthma attacks with difficulty in breathing, and wheezing. Over a period of time the attacks tend to get more frequent in this type of child, and it is also noticed that he is not completely well between attacks. He will have some wheeze on most days, and will often wake at night and cough or wheeze. In many children of this type there are no longer definite asthma attacks separated by periods of good health, but instead the child has continuous asthma which varies in severity from day to day. Obviously he is likely to miss a good deal of schooling and to be limited in his everyday activities. Because of the troublesome nature of the asthma, treatment is often needed more or less continuously and powerful drugs such as cromoglycate (Intal) or steroids will often be used. Although 80 per cent of children with this type of asthma begin to have trouble before the age of 4 years it must be remembered that they only form a small part of all the children who have symptoms as young as this and not all asthmatics are going to develop into this troublesome type. Experience suggests that boys who have bad infantile eczema and develop definite attacks of asthma before the age of 3 years are more likely to have troublesome asthma later, but there are no hard and fast rules.

Asthma in Older Children

Most parents of young asthmatic children are concerned about how the condition may affect the development of their child and whether or not it will clear up. In a disease which can last for many years, during which time the child will often change his doctor a number of times, it is naturally very difficult to be sure about the answers to such questions. A very different picture of asthma is obtained by looking at children who need to attend hospital and those who are managed in general practice, because the hospital group are likely to be rather more severely affected. Perhaps the most useful figures are those obtained by asking large numbers of school-children about their medical histories irrespective of whether or not they have required treatment. Such studies have been carried out a number of times and results from Britain, Australia and the United States agree that about 60 per cent of children with asthma will have stopped wheezing by the age of 10 years and about 80 to 90 per cent by the age of 13 to 14 years. Again it is not possible to predict which child will grow out of his asthma earlier and which later, nor to predict which children will continue to wheeze after puberty. The popular myth that the asthma either clears up at the age of 7 or 14 years is just not true. The general picture is very encouraging because the vast majority of children with asthma do grow out of it as they get older and this has no relation to the severity of the asthma—a bad asthmatic has just as good a chance of growing out of it as a mild one. The fact that most children will eventually lose their symptoms makes it very important to ensure that they have the very best treatment while they are still having attacks, so that they may eventually be left with healthy lungs. Unfortunately, there has been some tendency in the past to undertreat asthmatic children because "they will grow out of it anyway".

The pattern of asthma in the older children is usually one of decreasing severity and frequency of attacks until eventually they seem to stop. Even after "growing out" of the asthma, the child may have a tendency to wheeze a little from time to time, and this can be shown up by an exercise test years after the at-

The Patterns of Asthma in Children

tacks have stopped. This shows that the child is still basically the same person (his inherited characteristics have not changed) but his bronchial tubes have stopped reacting so easily. Some children do continue to have their asthma just as badly as they get older and never lose it. A few more lose their asthma as children only to have it return later on as adults. Sometimes the asthma only begins in the later part of childhood and in that case it usually continues through puberty. But parents should remember that 9 out of 10 asthmatic children have every chance of losing their asthma as they grow older.

One of the greatest concerns of the parents of the asthmatic child is whether or not the disease will permanently damage the child's lungs even if he grows out of it. In its usual form asthma only involves the narrowing of the bronchial tubes from time to time and this causes temporary increases of lung volume and disturbances of the mixing of gas and blood. Unlike chronic bronchitis in adults, there is no repeated infection and damage to the walls of the bronchial tubes and, unlike emphysema, there is no breaking down of the lung tissue itself. The temporary nature of asthma can easily be demonstrated in the majority of asthmatic children because their lung function tests (which will be discussed later) return to normal between attacks. This never happens in chronic bronchitis, emphysema, or other diseases which cause damage to the lungs. All the evidence suggests that even the most severe type of childhood asthmatic has a good chance of ending up with normal lungs. Of course the asthmatic should never smoke and it is vital to impress this upon children since the habit is learnt from parents and school friends at a very early age. Any bronchitis caused by smoking will make the asthma worse and may hinder the return of lung function to normal. Occasionally the asthma may be associated with small areas of collapse of a lung and this can persist if not treated, and there are also very rare forms of asthma which are associated with lung damage. However, the most encouraging fact for the doctor treating asthmatic children is that almost all of his patients will have lost their asthma and have normal lungs by the time they leave his care.

Status Asthmaticus

A very severe attack of asthma which does not respond to regular treatment is usually called "status asthmaticus". It can occur in children with any of the types of asthma already described and does not occur exclusively in very "bad" cases. An attack of status asthmaticus usually begins like any other attack but for one reason or another it does not seem to settle down with the child's usual treatment. Over a period of hours or days the difficulty in breathing persists and the child may become very tired because of all the work he has to do in order to get the air in and out. Because of the poor mixing of gas and blood in his lungs he may not take up enough oxygen into his blood and this causes him to look blue—"cyanosed".

One of the problems about status asthmaticus is that the child becomes unresponsive to ordinary drugs and he may then take them in very large quantities in order to try to get some effect. The consumption of large amounts of bronchodilator drugs, especially from pressurized aerosol inhalers, can be dangerous in this situation and an increased death rate in children was seen when these inhalers were first introduced. Most children with status asthmaticus are admitted to hospital nowadays and respond rapidly to intensive treatment, especially with the steroid type of drug. It is very rare for a really life-threatening situation to develop if effective treatment is begun early on. This is one reason why the importance of childhood asthma should not be underestimated by parents or doctors, since a status attack is possible in almost any patient.

The Patterns of Asthma in Children

Ocassionally children die of asthma, but the death rate (mortality) should not be exaggerated. There are about three quarters of a million children with asthma at any one time in the United Kingdom and about 3 million in the United States. The death rate from asthma in children varies a bit but is around 50 per year in Britain. This means that 1 child with asthma dies each year for every 14,000 children with asthma who live in Britain. From these figures it can be seen that death from asthma is a very rare event indeed and 14 times more children are killed every year on the roads. This does not mean that we can sit back and relax because every death is a terrible tragedy. We must make sure that the best treatment is available for asthmatic children and that they, their parents and their doctors understand the nature of the disease.

CHAPTER 4

Investigating the Asthmatic Child

Almost every child with asthma will need medical attention at some time and in most cases this will be from his family doctor, who will examine him and arrange appropriate treatment. A smaller number of children with troublesome asthma will be referred to hospital for specialist investigation. This chapter will describe the sort of investigations which can be used to obtain a good understanding of a child attending a modern children's asthma clinic.

Consultations in the Clinic

At the heart of all medical investigations is the clinical interview in which the patient is asked to describe his illness and he is examined for signs of disease. Asthma is no exception to this rule and it is especially important to obtain a very clear and detailed history of the child's illness. Of course this is complicated in children by the fact that the history has to be obtained "second-hand" from the parents (usually the mother) rather than directly from the patient. The way in which the mother recounts the history will inevitably be biased by what she believes to be the problem or by what she has been told by other doctors or laymen. It is common, for example, for a mother to say that her child is allergic to cats and when asked how she knows this, for her to reply that the last doctor told her so because of a positive skin test to cat fur. In this example the mother would then be asked if she herself had noticed that the

Investigating the Asthmatic Child

child had become ill regularly on contact with cats and, unless he had, the story would not be accepted as important. When the mother is frightened, confused or angry she will often allow her feelings consciously or unconsciously to affect her answers to questions, and the doctor will need to understand this.

Parents often feel that all they will have to do is to recount some details of their child's asthma and they are surprised when they are then asked a whole lot more questions by the doctor. But asthma cannot be studied in isolation and it is essential to know as much as possible about the child, including his early development, his general health and previous illnesses, and his emotional state. In addition, it is important to find out as much as possible about the frequency and severity of his attacks and how much they are interfering with his every-day life. It will also be necessary to ask about asthma or related illnesses in the family and to take careful note of factors such as allergy, weather, exercise or infection which can influence his attacks. A great deal can be learned about the nature of the child's asthma by noting his response to different forms of treatment and the parents will be asked to give a detailed account of the medicines he has received previously and their effects, whether good or bad. All these questions will help the doctor to gain a better understanding of the disease and parents should appreciate that they are necessary, even if they may cause some embarrassment when they concern personal relationships within the family.

The child will normally be given a full physical examination on his first attendance at the clinic to assess his asthma and to make sure that there is nothing else obviously affecting him. Many people believe that a doctor can tell all there is to know about a patient simply by taking his pulse or listening to his chest, but in the case of asthma this could not be further from the truth. It will be recalled that a cardinal feature of asthma is that it varies so much from day to day and it is quite common for the child to be perfectly well on the day that he attends the clinic. In this case the doctor will find nothing abnormal on examination. Even if the child is wheezy when he is seen, the doctor only hears what everyone else can hear, even though it is through a stethoscope. Of course, the examination can give some idea about the general level of airways obstruction and the effect it is having on the child's health, but it rarely provides as much information as a careful history taken from the parents. Chronic and severe asthma in a child tends to cause some loss of normal growth and the child should be weighed and measured each time he attends the clinic. It can also cause some deformity of the rib cage and the doctor will be looking for any signs of this. Occasionally, a child is referred to the clinic with what appears to be asthma but is in fact something else. One of the chief functions of the examination is to make sure that this does not escape unnoticed.

Consultations in the clinic will be repeated as often as the condition of the child indicates. In some cases a single visit will be all that is needed, but other children will require more detailed investigations. The child with chronic, persistent asthma will often attend at intervals so that his progress can be followed during treatment. Very close cooperation is needed between the clinic doctor and the family doctor when planning the treatment of the child and supervising his progress, and each should be kept fully informed of any changes recommended by the other. Parents should never be shy of discussing their child with either doctor, nor of complaining if they are not happy with his progress, because more is learned about the asthmatic child in this way than by almost any other means.

Diary Cards

Because of the importance of documenting the progress of the child as accurately as possible, it is now quite common for

Investigating the Asthmatic Child

parents to be asked to keep a daily record of symptoms. This is usually best done with the help of a simple diary card, such as that illustrated in Fig. 4. Each evening the column for the day is filled in, providing information about the previous night and any daytime symptoms. In addition, the card is provided with

			DAYS			
			1	2	3	4
	(1) NIGHT	Good night... 0 Slept well but slightly wheezy or some coughing ... 1 Woken x 2-3 because of wheeze or cough ... 2 Bad night, awake most of time.. ... 3				
DAY TIME	(2) WHEEZE	None.. 0 Little . 1 Moderately bad ... 2 Severe ... 3				
	(3) ACTIVITY	Quite normal ... 0 Can run short distance... 1 Limited to walking . 2 Off school or indoors ... 3				
	(4) COUGH	None.. 0 Occasional .. 1 Frequent ... 2				
	(5) SPUTUM Add "Y" if yellow	None.. 0 Less than 3 tsps. = a little ... 1 More than 3 tsps. = a lot . 2				
		DAILY TOTAL ...				
	(6) FLOW METER READING	Before breakfast medicines ... a.m. Before bedtime medicines ... p.m.				
	(7) DRUGS (Record number of times given each day)	Name and dose ...				
	(8) COMMENTS	(Only if there is anything unusual to report)				

Fig. 4. Part of the diary card used to follow the progress of the child day by day. On each day a number is placed in the appropriate box, to indicate how the child has been over the previous 24 hours. For example, if the previous night had been perfectly good, 0 would be placed in the top box, and if during the day he had had a moderate amount of wheeze a 2 would be placed in the second box down and so on. When the child is provided with a peak flow meter to measure his breathing at home, the numbers are placed in the box provided. The number of doses of each drug taken is also written down in the box labelled "Drugs". Any additional comments, for example if a child had measles, are written at the bottom of the chart. (Reprinted from Connolly and Godfrey, Journal of Asthma Research, 1970)

a very important section in which the number of doses of any medicines actually taken are recorded. The use of this type of diary card has a number of important advantages. In the first place it is always difficult to give an accurate summary of the child's condition over a period of time such as with monthly clinic visits, and it is normal for the parents to be particularly influenced by the child's condition in the few days before the appointment. The diary serves as a more correct record over the whole month and is used to help both the parents and the doctors to build up a true picture of the child.

Another important use of the diary is the information it can provide on the amount of treatment that the child needs and this can also serve as a check on the symptoms recorded in the diary by the mother. The record may alert the doctor to the fact that the mother is tending to underestimate her child's complaints because there are few symptoms scores and yet he is using a lot of medicines. Equally, it can help the doctor to judge the value of a treatment; for example, if a child is supposed to be well controlled by a particular drug and yet his diary shows that he is frequently needing to take additional medications, then the effectiveness of the drug may be questioned. The diary card shown in Fig. 4 is also provided with an additional section in which the parents can record the results of the simple breathing tests carried out at home which will be described later. It is particularly helpful to compare the results of these measurements with the symptoms and drug consumption, all recorded over a month in the one diary.

It would be rather tedious to use a daily diary card for months or years on end, and they are mostly used for the assessment of the child during his first month or two of attendance at the clinic, or when he is being stabilized on a new type of treatment. During these times of evaluation, the diary is a convenient way of making monthly clinic interviews almost as good as daily interviews.

X-ray and Blood Tests

When patients attend a hospital clinic with a chest complaint they usually expect to have a chest X-ray and some blood tests, and of course these are often necessary. Children are naturally very scared of blood tests (and sometimes even of X-rays) because they believe that they will hurt them. This fear is not helped by the occasional unwise parent who has threatened to "take the child to the doctor for a blood test" when he has been naughty in the past. Nor is it helped by the occasional doctor who is not particularly good at blood tests in small children and takes longer over the test as a result. For these reasons, most specialists who are used to dealing with children take as few blood tests as possible and often avoid taking any at all during the first visit of the child to the clinic when he is likely to be especially afraid.

An X-ray of the chest will normally be carried out for any new patient attending an asthma clinic unless the child has already had one recently. The X-ray tells us very little about the asthma itself because it is impossible to see the obstruction of the tiny bronchial tubes on the film and all that is found during an attack is that the lungs appear unduly full of air. The main reason for taking an X-ray is to be sure that the child does not also have some other type of chest disease such as tuberculosis or cystic fibrosis, though these conditions are very rare. Infections can often cause the asthmatic child to have an attack and so it is also usual to take a chest X-ray during a particularly bad attack to find out if he has pneumonia which would need treating.

Blood tests are used to measure very many different aspects of the functions of the body. Like X-rays they are not of very great help in the management of the average asthmatic child, but are used chiefly to check on other possible problems such as anaemia or infection. Asthmatic children usually have an increased number of blood cells called eosinophils and an increased concentration of the protein called IgE, both of which have something to do with allergic reactions. Unfortunately, it has not been possible to use these or any other blood tests to predict the severity of the child's asthma nor to plan the best kind of treatment.

During a very severe attack of asthma which needs admission to hospital, an entirely different type of blood test may be needed to tell how the child is responding to treatment. This test is to measure the concentrations of oxygen, carbon dioxide and acid in the arterial blood. The skin over an artery at the wrist or in front of the elbow is first anaesthetized with a small injection and then a sample of arterial blood is drawn into a syringe using a fine needle. Since the blood in the arteries is under high pressure, it is necessary for the doctor or a nurse to press on the puncture site for a few minutes afterwards. When carried out in this way, arterial puncture is as painless and safe as the ordinary type of blood test in which the sample is collected from a vein. The information obtained from the arterial puncture in the very sick child is helpful in deciding what drugs should be used and whether or not he needs to be in an oxygen tent.

Allergy Tests

The investigation of possible allergies is important for a full understanding of a child's asthma because of the clues that it may provide for prevention or treatment of attacks. Most people think of allergy tests simply in terms of skin tests to a whole variety of substances, but this type of testing is useless in isolation and there are also a number of other allergy tests which may be used from time to time. It was pointed out in the previous chapter that one of the most important parts of allergic investigation is the history taken from the child or his

Investigating the Asthmatic Child

parents about the relationship between his attacks and contact with things (allergens) to which it is thought he is allergic. Great care is needed to avoid putting ideas into the family's mind and to make sure that the suspected allergen really does cause an attack every time that the child meets it and that the attacks are not just coincidental.

In addition to a history about possible allergies, it is useful to test the child to a number of substances which are commonly associated with allergic diseases. There are several ways of doing this but the simplest, and in many ways the best, is by skin testing. In the usual type of skin test, a small drop of each of the test substances is placed on the child's forearm and each drop is then pricked into the skin with a separate needle to avoid mixing the substances with each other. It is not really fair to call this "pricking" because only the very outermost layer of skin is gently lifted with the needle tip and this is completely painless, so that the test is possible in even young children. Within a few minutes of the test a positive reaction is shown up by a small, white, itching bump appearing which may be surrounded by some reddening of the skin (Fig. 5). The intensity of the allergy is related to the size of the bump, but even the most severe reactions in this type of test go down over half an hour or so and leave no after effects. Almost every asthmatic child will have at least one or two positive reactions and they often have several. Unless the substance under test has also been noticed to cause the child to wheeze regularly, the the positive test just shows that he produces (harmless) allergic antibodies in his blood more easily than usual.

Occasionally slightly different types of skin test are needed in asthmatic patients which may cause the same early reaction but also produce a rather larger swelling some hours later. This type of late reaction is very rare in children. Some doctors prefer to inject the test substances into the skin with a syringe rather than by the prick tests described above. There is really

Your Child With Asthma

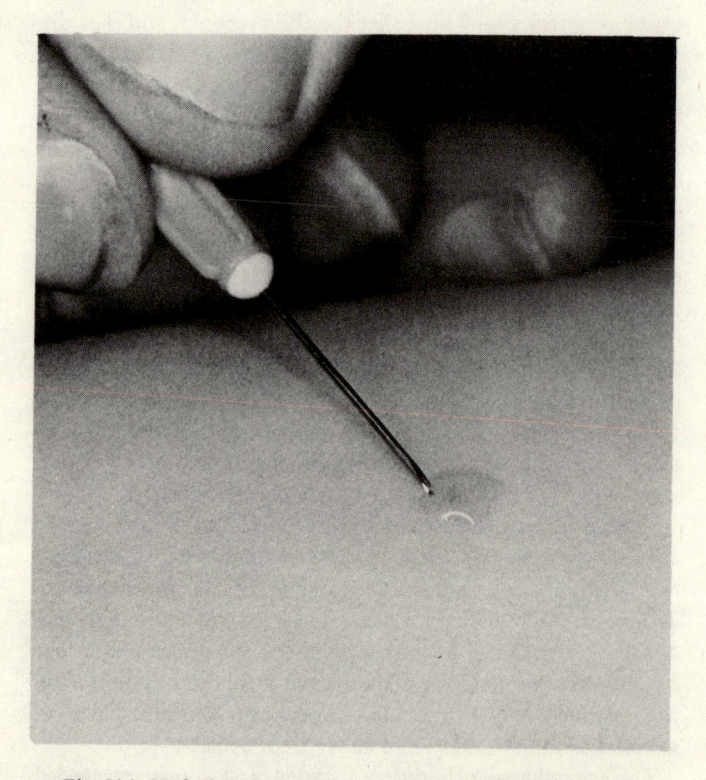

Fig. 5(a). Method used to prick a very small amount of solution into the skin when testing for allergy. The needle is used to gently raise the outermost portion of skin, so that it does not even draw blood and the process is almost painless.

Investigating the Asthmatic Child

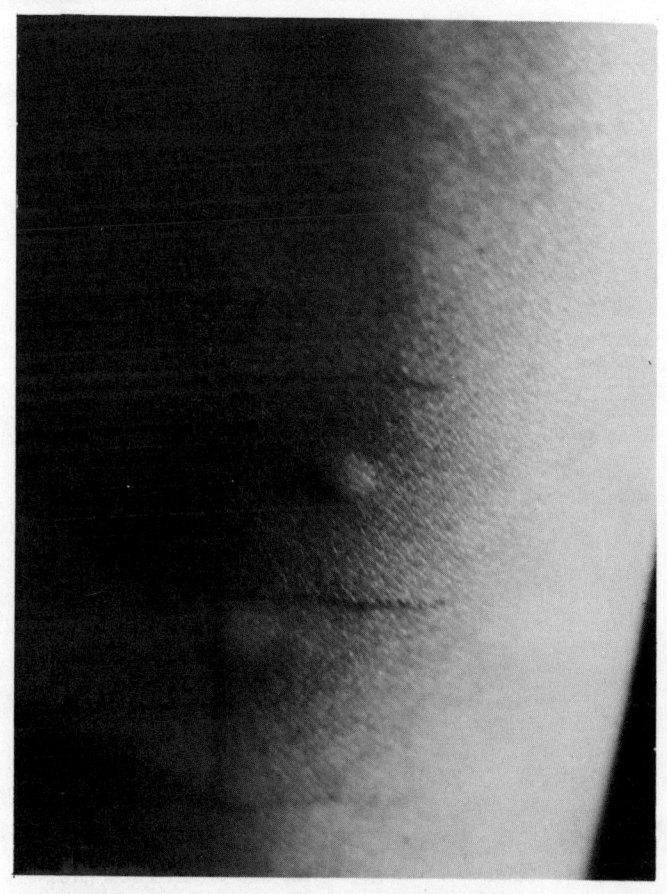

(b) A positive skin test showing a small swelling at the site where the substance was pricked into the skin.

no advantage in this method now and almost all doctors dealing with children use the prick test which is less frightening. Another type of skin test which may cause confusion is used to test whether or not the child has been in contact with tuberculosis. This has nothing to do with the asthma but is often used during the initial screening of the child. It is carried out either by pricking the solution into the skin with a special gun (Heaft Test) or by injecting it with a syringe (Mantoux Test). The Heaf test is generally preferred for routine use because it is less painful.

In some hospitals tests are also carried out to find out if the child has a decrease in his lung function when he breathes in substances to which he is thought to be allergic. These bronchial challenge tests as they are called are not used very often because they can be rather difficult to carry out and take a lot of time. They are very useful for the occasional child whose asthma can be shown to be caused by inhaling just one or two substances and nothing else so that desensitization treatment is really worthwhile. Parents should realize that doctors who are very interested in the allergic side of the asthma story might well spend more time on these types of test than on some of the others described in this chapter.

Lung Function Tests

Asthma is a disease which causes symptoms by altering the function of the lungs in a very fluctuating manner. It would seem very logical to judge the severity of the asthma by tests which measure lung function and yet there are very many asthmatic children who have never had a single test of their lung function. The reason is that some doctors believe that children will not be able to do the tests properly and others do not really understand the tests themselves. In reality the tests are simple, painless, very useful, and children generally carry

Investigating the Asthmatic Child

them out excellently.

Since the chief functional problem in asthma is obstruction of the bronchial tubes (airways obstruction—*see* Chapter 1), the lung function tests that are most useful are those which measure the resistance to flow of air through the tubes. The simplest test of all, and probably the most useful test of all, is called the Peak Flow Rate (PEF). In this test the child is asked to take a full breath in and then to blow out as fast as he possibly can through a clock-like meter which measures the maximum speed that he can expel his breath. This test is illustrated in Fig. 6. If the child has airways obstruction, he can-

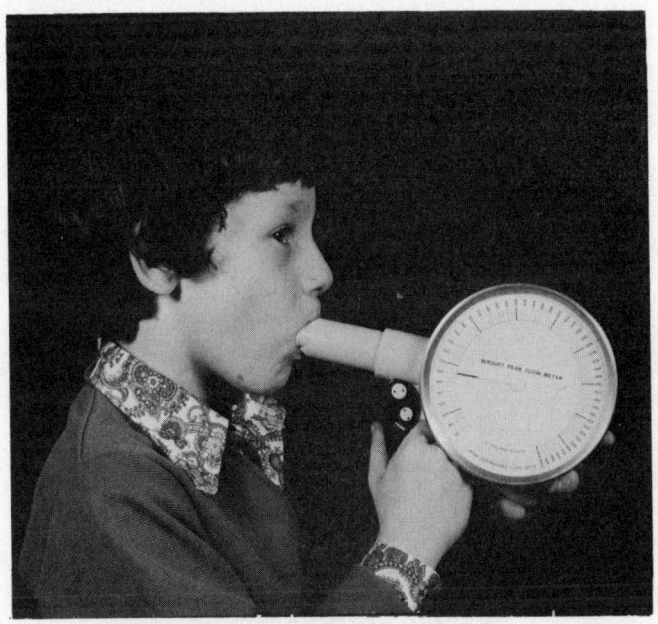

Fig. 6. Child performing a breathing test using peak flow meter. After a full breath he blows out as fast as he can and the speed which he reaches is indicated on the dial of the meter.

Your Child With Asthma

not achieve as great a speed as normal and so his PEF will be reduced. The peak flow meter is a very handy machine for children to be given to use at home and it was mentioned above that this may be a useful way of measuring his performance in his home surroundings as compared to the hospital. There is quite a wide variation in the normal range of PRF and parents should not be unduly worried by low values recorded at home if their child is otherwise quite well.

For some purposes it is helpful to have a rather more accurate measure of airways obstruction and a simple machine called a spirometer is then used (*see* Fig. 7). The child takes a

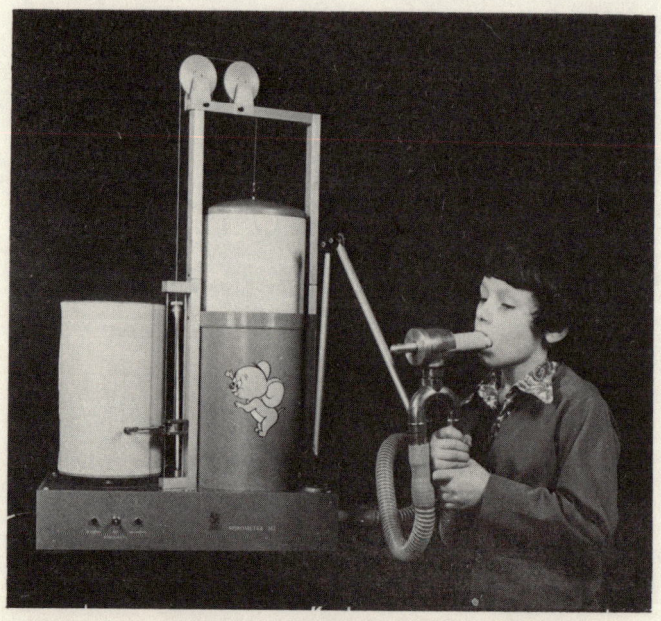

Fig. 7. Child performing a breathing test with a machine which records the size of his breaths and the amount of air that he can blow out as fast as possible in one second.

Investigating the Asthmatic Child

deep breath in and then blows out through the tubing as fast and as long as he can. The machine produces a record on paper of the volume of air he breathes out and this is used to calculate the amount expired in the first second ($FEV_{1\,sec}$) and the total "vital capacity" expired (FVC). Obviously when a child has airways obstruction he cannot breathe out so fast and the volume expired in the first second is reduced. This type of test is less dependent on the effort of the patient and little more reliable than the peak flow rate, but the information that it gives is really quite similar.

Occasionally it is useful to be able to measure the airways resistance and volume of air in the lungs very accurately, either to help in the management of the child or for the purposes of research into the causes and treatment of asthma. These measurements can be made with the help of a machine called a "whole body plethysmograph". This is just a small chamber in which the child sits and breathes through tubing containing a device which measures the flow of gas in and out of his mouth. By measuring the air pressure in the chamber and at the child's mouth, it is possible to calculate the resistance and lung volume. Although this machine sounds very complicated, it is quite simple for the patient and does not involve anything other than panting in and out of a tube for a few breaths.

Exercise Tests

A very common complaint of children with asthma is that they become wheezy when they take certain types of exercise, especially after running. It is possible to take advantage of this feature to study the child's asthma by arranging to measure his lung function before and after a period of exercise. The best way to carry out this test is to have the child run fairly hard for about 6 minutes either back and forth along a corridor or on a treadmill running machine and to measure his peak flow rate before, during and after the exercise. In this test the asthmatic will actually improve a little during the early part of the run but will begin to wheeze towards the end and become really quite wheezy for the first 3 or 4 minutes after stopping the run. This wheeze then passes off rapidly and is usually completely gone after about half an hour, or sooner if some treatment is given. The particular value of the exercise test is that it produces the reaction described in almost every asthmatic child, even when they are otherwise completely well, and it does not produce the reaction in healthy children or children with other diseases. This means that when there is some doubt about the diagnosis, the doctor can carry out an exercise test and if the child produces the typical response then it is virtually certain that he has asthma. This is especially helpful when the child is otherwise completely fit between attacks when he attends the clinic.

Exercise tests can also be used to gain some idea about the likely severity of the child's asthma, and, even more important, to test the effectiveness of various drugs used to treat the asthma. Most of the drugs which are used to relieve attacks will also prevent the child from wheezing if they are given before the exercise test. By carrying out the exercise test on two occasions, once after treatment with the drug to be investigated and once after an inactive, dummy drug which looks the same, it is possible to measure the degree of protection given by the real drug compared with the dummy. The exercise test really just produces a short, sharp, "mini" attack of asthma under controlled conditions in the laboratory and provides a very convenient way of investigating the asthmatic child.

Psychological Tests

It has been pointed out before that emotional factors can be very important in provoking attacks in the asthmatic child, and

Investigating the Asthmatic Child

like allergy, infection and physical factors, the emotional component also needs to be investigated. Of course the great majority of asthmatic children do not have any intellectual or personality problems and only a few will need serious psychiatric treatment. However, the normal, healthy fears and anxieties of the child may well be making his asthma worse and it is as well for the doctor to know about this. Some parents resent the suggestion that their child should undergo psychological testing because they think that this implies he is disturbed, but of course this is not at all correct. Children with asthma have a rather higher level of intelligence on average and do not suffer from mental illness any more often than other children. The purpose of psychological testing is to provide information on the way that normal emotional reactions might be influencing the course of the child's illness and to give a guide for treatment.

Psychological tests are usually carried out by a Clinical Psychologist who is not often a medical doctor but who has had special training in psychology and particularly in children's problems. The tests generally consist of a series of written or spoken problems which the child is asked to complete, which have been specially designed and tested in large numbers of normal children. There are also questionnaires which the parents and sometimes the schoolteacher are asked to complete about the child's personality and behaviour. In most cases the Clinical Psychologist will also interview one or both parents in an informal way to supplement the information obtained from the tests. All the information is, of course, confidential and is treated in exactly the same way as other parts of the child's medical records.

* * *

It can be seen from this chapter that there are a considerable number of useful investigations which can be carried out in children with asthma. Not every test is needed in every case, and some clinics and hospitals will not even be able to undertake them all. The type of test used will depend to some extent upon the personal views of the doctor seeing the child, but so long as the best interests of the child are always kept in mind the end result of the investigations will be a better understanding of the problem.

CHAPTER 5

The Treatment of the Asthmatic Child

Parents of asthmatic children are naturally concerned that their child should receive the best possible treatment and they are often confused by the different methods which may be tried. This reflects to some extent the differing opinions within the medical profession and the fact that the treatment of asthma is one of the most rapidly changing fields of medicine. In recent years there has been great improvement in some of the standard types of drugs which can be used and entirely new drugs have also been developed, mainly in the United Kingdom. In addition, a much clearer understanding of the place of allergic, physical and emotional treatment is being developed. This chapter is not designed as a parents "do it yourself" guide to treatment of asthma, but rather to explain the reasons why different forms of treatment are tried and how they are thought to work. The ultimate decision on which treatment to use must rest with the doctor actually in charge of the case.

Which Asthmatic Children Need Treatment?

Asthma is a very common condition in childhood, but only a very small proportion of asthmatic children, perhaps one in five, will need more than the occasional simple drug. It is probable that most asthmatics never come to the attention of doctors at all, or have attacks that are so mild that they do not need any treatment. At the other extreme are children whose asthma is so troublesome that they need more or less continuous treatment to enable them to get on with their normal lives. It is worth briefly reviewing the problems which may cause parents or doctors to believe that a child needs treatment for his asthma.

Wheezing is very common in babies but the vast majority of wheezy babies do not grow up to become asthmatic children, even though they may still need treatment at the time. In fact, the drugs which are so effective in asthmatic children have very little action on the wheezy baby and treatment consists largely of careful attention to his food and fluid requirements and occasionally using an oxygen tent.

Most children with asthma who need regular treatment are between about 4 and 14 years old and of course most of them have it very mildly. This type of child may get one or two attacks a year, often associated with an infection, and the wheezing may last just for a few hours or a day. It is helpful to have some simple medicine at home for children like this because their wheezing can usually be stopped quite easily and they may not even need to see a doctor. Some children who only have occasional attacks are more severely affected and the attack lasts longer. Although they may be helped by simple treatment, they sometimes require more powerful drugs and it is usually necessary for them to see the doctor.

The asthmatic children who give their parents greatest concern are those with very frequent asthma, whether it is mild or severe. The asthma can easily interfere with their ordinary activities or schooling unless it is treated effectively. Because every child does not respond in the same way it is usually necessary to try different treatments very carefully to get the best results. This type of child will need fairly regular medical supervision by his family doctor and often by the hospital, but once he is on a good regime he will only need to attend occasionally.

As the child grows older, the asthma becomes less severe in almost all cases, and the interval between attacks gets longer. Eventually the child finds that he no longer needs to take any regular treatment. This is one of the most encouraging aspects of childhood asthma.

Allergic and Environmental Treatment

Because asthmatic children are so often allergic subjects a great deal of effort has been put in to devising treatments to reduce their sensitivities. Some doctors are very enthusiastic about this type of treatment but its real value in the individual child needs careful assessment, especially since there are now such effective drugs available.

One of the best ways of dealing with allergic asthma is to avoid the substance (allergen) which is causing the problem. If the child is trully allergic to the cat and wheezes every time they are in the same room, then the cat should go, but if the association is not so clear then the emotional harm of loosing the pet could be worse than the possible allergic benefit. In general, it is unwise for asthmatic children to keep furry pets because they may become allergic to them or the dust that they carry; fish or reptiles are more acceptable! A particular problem is that almost all asthmatic children are allergic to house dust, or more correctly to the tiny mite which lives in the dust. This mite is especially common in the dust in and around beds and it is often helpful to try to reduce this to a minimum. To some extent the trouble taken over avoiding house dust should be a matter of trial and error, with parents noting whether or not the child improves. Common sense precautions include vacuum cleaning carpets, curtains and bed-clothes regularly when the child is not in the room, using foam rather than feather pillows, and putting the mattress in a thin plastic sheet to prevent dust getting in or out of it. Stricter precautions against house dust are only justified in the rare child for whom it can be proved beyond doubt that this is the major cause of his troubles.

When it is impossible to avoid an allergen which is definitely contributing to the asthma, then it is reasonable to try to desensitize the child to the substance in question. A good example of this is pollen asthma which causes some children to wheeze for a short period of the year when the particular pollen to which they are allergic is in the air. The principle behind desensitization is that the child is given very dilute injections of the pollen and he builds up resistance against it. The strength of the injections is increased in steps until the child has acquired enough resistance so that even if he breathes in the pollen he does not wheeze. This type of desensitization treatment is commonly used in asthma, especially in North America, and the child may be given injections against a whole variety of different substances at the same time. It must be admitted that there is very little scientific proof that such unselective treatment does any good for the vast majority of asthmatic children. The child is usually allergic to many known and unknown substances so that desensitization cannot be complete, and in any case he is also provoked into an attack by other factors such as infection, exercise or emotion against which the desensitization is useless. Hay fever is usually helped by desensitization injections so that some asthmatics who have both hay fever and asthma may feel much better after treatment, but this is really due to the improvement in the hay fever. Against the possible value of desensitization must be set the inconvenience of annual courses of injections which children do not like, and the fact that the injection may sometimes provoke an attack itself, so that the patient should always have some treatment at hand when having his injection.

The Treatment of the Asthmatic Child

Doctors are tending to move away from the policy of giving injections against a large number of substances merely on the basis of a positive skin test. Much more attention is now paid to the relationship between observations by patient or parents, skin tests, and lung function tests after inhaling or eating the suspected allergen. If this information suggests that the patient really is having asthma because of allergy to something which cannot easily be avoided, then a course of desensitization injections will usually be recommended, and they may have to be repeated each year for several years.

Parents sometimes move home because they believe that their child will be better in a different environment. It has been pointed out in Chapter 2 that any improvement may be due to a whole variety of factors rather than just to the change in air. There is no doubt that some asthmatic children are genuinely better in a different climate, but this is very much an individual matter. Family life should not be disrupted by moving home unless it can be shown beyond all doubt that this is the only solution after all other effective forms of treatment have been tried. The question of special schools is considered later on.

Drug Treatment

Almost all asthmatic children will need to be treated with drugs at some time. There are several different drugs with similar actions and a number of different groups of drug each working in its own way. Quite often it is useful to combine one or more types of treatment at the same time and this means that there is really a large number of different possibilities to offer. In this section the main groups of drugs will be described to give the parent an idea of their place in the management of asthmatic children and the possible problems resulting from their use.

(a) *Drugs which relax the bronchial tubes-bronchodilators*

The bronchodilator drugs are the simplest and probably the most useful of all drugs used to treat asthmatic children. They act on the muscles surrounding the bronchial tubes and cause them to relax so that the tubes widen and the child's breathing becomes easier. Many of these drugs act by imitating the body's own reaction to stress, which is to activate the sympathetic nervous system, and so this type of drug is called a "-sympathomimetic" drug. For a long time the only drugs of any use in asthma were the sympathomimetics, particularly ephedrine given by mouth and adrenaline (epinephrine in the U.S.A.) given by injection. Unfortunately these drugs mimic many of the body's stress reactions, including effects on the heart such as making it beat faster. In an effort to improve on this type of treatment, sympathomimetic drugs were developed which were inhaled by the patient so that they acted directly on the lung. The most popular drug of this type for a long time was isoprenaline (isoproterenol in the U.S.A.) and it is certainly very effective. However, it also causes the heart to beat faster, and there has been some evidence to suggest that it can be dangerous when taken too often. This can easily occur if a child is given a pressurized aerosol can of the drug to carry around and is not supervized closely. More recently, a number of drugs have been developed which have the beneficial effects of sympathomimetics as far as the lungs are concerned, but do not have the unwanted effects on the heart. These selective drugs, such as orciprenaline or salbutamol, can be given by mouth or by aerosol and are now being developed for use by injection as well.

The sympathomimetic drugs are ideal for treating the wheezy child because they are effective and act very quickly. They are probably the only type of treatment that will be needed by the majority of asthmatic children who only have oc-

The Treatment of the Asthmatic Child

casional mild attacks, but it is important that they are given in an adequate dose and begun early enough before the attack really has a chance to develop too much. In the more severely affected child these drugs may have to be given more often or even continuously, and in the most troublesome types of asthma they are not very effective. Nowadays most doctors would prescribe one of the modern, selective bronchodilators to be taken by mouth which are quite safe and do not affect the heart rate. In an emergency the child is often given an injection of adrenaline (epinephrine) because this is still the most powerful and suitable drug in this situation. The inhalation of bronchodilators from pressurized aerosols is not usually recommended for children because of the possibility that the child may use it too much if he is allowed to carry the inhaler with him. There is, however, no doubt that this type of treatment, especially with the safer selective drugs, can be very useful for quick relief of symptoms at night or when brought on by exercise and so some parents or older children may well be given an aerosol to keep handy. Parents are sometimes worried that their child may become addicted to the drugs he is taking, but none of these drugs cause the mental addiction that occurs with narcotics of some other agents and the child is easily able to stop the treatment when his asthma improves.

There is another group of bronchodilator drug which acts in a slightly different way to the sympathomimetics but which has a similar overall effect. The commonest drug in this group is called aminophylline and this is given by injection for emergencies, or as a suppository to be absorbed from the rectum. Although suppositories are obviously rather unpleasant to use, this is quite an effective way of treating an acute attack, especially at night or when the child is vomiting and cannot keep down his usual drugs. There are also preparations of this type of drug which can be taken by mouth and these are quite popular in some areas. This group is sometimes combined with the sympathomimetic group in one tablet which the makers claim is better than either type of drug alone. There is really no scientific evidence to support this idea and most specialists prefer not to give combined tablets.

(b) *Drugs to prevent attacks occurring—"Intal"*

In 1967 the discovery of a new drug was announced and it has turned out to be one of the most important advances ever made in the treatment of troublesome childhood asthma. This drug has the official name of sodium cromoglycate in Britain and cromolyn sodium in the U.S.A. It is more commonly known by its trade names of Intal, Lomudal or Aerane. The importance of this drug is that it strengthens the cells in the body which contain chemicals that cause the bronchial tubes to constrict. In the presence of Intal, these cells do not break down if an allergic reaction occurs or even if the child takes some exercise, and so he does not wheeze. If the chemicals have already liberated from their cells, then Intal can have no effect and so it is of no help once the child is actually wheezing. For this reason, Intal and other similar drugs which are being developed are preventative or prophylactic agents rather than improving agents such as the bronchodilators described above.

Because it prevents attacks but has no effect once an attack is in progress, Intal has to be given continuously every day even while the child is free from wheeze. In fact, the drug is only doing its job if the child is not having attacks. This means that Intal is only used for children who have asthma so frequently that it is worth taking treatment every day to prevent attacks rather than to use other drugs to treat the attacks which develop. The ideal child to treat with Intal is one who is having trouble from his asthma on more days or nights than he is well and who has the asthma all the year round.

The main disadvantage of Intal is that it is a powder which

The Treatment of the Asthmatic Child

has to be inhaled from a special type of inhaler and this requires some skill so that it may be difficult for the younger children. It is often possible to teach a 4-year-old to take the drug and there are even a few 2-year-olds who have used it successfully, but in general it is more suitable for older children. Another problem is that it probably needs to be taken at least 4 times daily for long periods and some parents and children find this difficult to arrange. It must also be appreciated that Intal does not work in every case and about 1 in 4 children will not get adequate control from the drug, even when combined with extra doses of bronchodilators or other drugs. If a child actually develops an attack while taking Intal, it becomes difficult for him to inhale the powder but he should continue to try because it may help him to recover more quickly. He will, of course, need to take other drugs at this time because Intal will not help the attack itself. Finally, although Intal has been shown to be an extremely safe drug over many years, it is only preventing attacks and not "curing" the asthma, so that the potential for bad attacks remains. This means that the child should remain under regular supervision by his doctor and should not start or stop the drug except under doctor's orders.

(c) *Drugs for severe asthma—the steroids*

The most powerful drugs used to treat asthma belong to the group that are called "steroids" because their basic chemical structure is based on the steroid nucleus. In the body there are many natural steroids which serve as messengers (hormones) regulating various aspects of normal function. Some of the most important steroid hormones are produced by the adrenal glands which lie adjacent to the kidneys, and it is these adrenal steroids which are of such interest in asthma, because of their ability to open up the airways. The most important of these adrenal hormones is called "cortisol" and the related drugs used in treatment are cortisone, prednisone, prednisolone, and betamethasone. All these steroids have a remarkable ability to relieve an asthmatic attack by actions on the bronchial tubes which are not fully understood even now, and they are the only effective drugs in the really severe attacks which are usually called "status asthmaticus".

The problem with adrenal steroids is that they also have a number of unwanted side effects which can be dangerous if they are used unwisely. The chief side effect as far as children are concerned is that they can reduce normal growth and cause them to be too short if they are given for long enough. Other side effects include putting on too much weight, rounding of the face ("moon face"), and occasionally loss of calcium from the bones or problems with control of the level of sugar in the blood. It is because of this rather awesome list of possible hazards that many doctors and parents are very unwilling for the asthmatic child to take these drugs and nobody would use them if other, simpler drugs could do the job. However, the steroids are undoubtedly the most effective of all drugs for treating asthma and may literally be life-saving in some cases. Because they are so important, a great deal of work has been done to find safer ways of using them and the artificial steroids such as prednisolone have been developed which have much less tendency to cause problems than the natural hormones. These steroids can be taken for a few days at a time every few weeks or so without causing any trouble and this is commonly used in children with infrequent but severe attacks. Another very important discovery was that steroids could be given safely as a single dose every other morning because in this way they did not disturb the body's own rise and fall of steroid levels. This form of treatment is useful in children who need the drugs for longer periods.

Part of the problem with steroids given to the child is that they can cause his adrenal glands to reduce the production of

The Treatment of the Asthmatic Child

their own steroids and this may be the reason for growth limitation. But even more important than the growth effect is the protection against stress, such as an infection or an operation, which the natural adrenal hormones provide. If they have been suppressed by treatment, then the child could be at some risk in a time of stress and would need extra amounts of steroid tablets or injections. For this reason, all parents and older children should know the importance of taking steroids and should keep a record of the name and dose of the drug. If they have been taken for more than a few days at a time, they should never be stopped suddenly without doctor's advice. This problem of adrenal suppression can be overcome by making the child's own adrenal glands produce the extra cortisol needed to treat his asthma. This is done by giving injections every few days of a drug called ACTH or Synacthen, which is itself a hormone whose normal function is to stimulate the adrenal glands to produce cortisol. Injections of ACTH have been used successfully for many years to treat childhood asthma with less side effects than other steroids, but it does mean giving frequent injections which children naturally do not like. In any case, giving prednisolone tablets every other morning is also very safe and usually gives adequate control of the asthma.

A major advance in steroid treatment of asthma occurred in 1969 when an entirely new type of steroid called beclomethasone dipropionate was developed in the U.K. This drug is inhaled from a pressurized aerosol and acts locally on the bronchial tubes. Although some of it escapes into the blood stream and reaches the adrenal glands, they are very insensitive to its effect and so it does not suppress them, nor does it stop the child growing. Recent trials of this drug in children with asthma have been very encouraging and it can apparently give good control of the asthma without the risk of side effects. The chief problem is that it has to be inhaled and so it is not suitable for the very young child (though at least one 2-year-old has taken it successfully) and it is not effective if the child is already so wheezy that he cannot inhale it properly. In this respect it resembles Intal, though of course it is an entirely different type of drug. It is most effective for the long-term treatment of the child who would otherwise wheeze every day and who is not controlled by Intal. If a child taking beclomethasone does become very wheezy he may need a few days of steroid tablets to tide him over and his doctor should be consulted.

A good deal of space has been devoted to the steroids because they are often feared and misunderstood by parents. There is no doubt that they must be treated with respect, but when used properly they can provide an excellent form of treatment. Doctors know how to avoid unwanted side effects in almost all cases, either by using alternate day treatment, ACTH injections, or nowadays by aerosol steroids. Steroids are not used unless they can do the job more rapidly or more effectively than other forms of treatment. In many cases the child concerned would be quite unable to live a normal life without steroids and by using them he is able to grow out of his asthma like other children with normal physical and mental development. In the most severe type of asthma which is discussed at the end of this chapter, steroids are often life-saving. The verdict as far as these drugs are concerned should really be "Respect—yes; Fear—no."

(d) *Antibiotics, antihistamines, etc.*

Many children treated with antibiotics such as penicillin or ampicillin when they have an attack of asthma, and parents are often impressed by the way they seem to respond. It must be clearly stated, however, that antibiotics have no action whatsoever on the bronchial tubes and are in no way responsible for

The Treatment of the Asthmatic Child

any improvement which occurs. The truth is that most attacks of asthma only last a day or two and so the child would have improved in any case and it is just a coincidence that he has been taking the antibiotic. It is quite hard for some parents, and even doctors, to accept these facts, but to ignore them does a disservice to the asthmatic child whose attack would pass off much more rapidly and completely if he were given one of the effective drugs discussed above.

It is not completely wrong to use antibiotics for asthma because the child can have an infection which also needs treating at the same time. Most infections which precipitate asthmatic attacks are caused by viruses and do not respond to antibiotics, but occasionally the child will have a bacterial infection which would respond. The final decision about antibiotics should rest with the doctor, who should use them together with appropriate anti-asthmatic treatment if he has good reason to believe that the child has a bacterial infection. Unfortunately, family doctors are often pressurized into using antibiotics by parents who have been led to expect that they will help the asthma. Excessive use of antibiotics means that there is the risk of developing drug-resistant types of bacteria which could present serious problems if a real infection occurred.

Another type of drug frequently used for asthmatic children belongs to the group of antihistamines which are widely used to treat such allergic diseases as hay fever and urticaria (hives), as well as sea-sickness. The original reason for trying these drugs in asthma was the mistaken belief that they would work because asthma is "an allergic disease". It has been shown that histamine has nothing to do with human asthma and so antihistamines do not relax the bronchial tubes. However, these drugs produce mild sedation and help to dry the bronchial tubes and so they have proved to be of some use in calming the restless child who has mild asthma, especially at night. If they are used in the daytime, they will make him sleepy and he will have poor concentration at school. Of course, if the child also has hay fever then antihistamines might be needed to control this symptom for its own sake. Many children with asthma have a lot of cough because of irritation of their bronchial tubes by the asthmatic process. It is common for cough mixtures to be prescribed but these have little effect, as most parents are aware. Cough mixtures often contain rather small amounts of a combination of bronchodilator, antihistamine and sedative; better results are usually obtained by giving the child full doses of a bronchodilator drug on its own.

Psychological and Physical Treatment

The importance of emotional factors in provoking asthma has been discussed in Chapter 2 and it was pointed out that, while only a small proportion of children are frankly disturbed, very many more have asthma which is influenced by their emotional state. For this reason there have been many attempts made to treat asthma by psychological methods and many exaggerated claims of success. One problem is that there are many different schools of thought amongst psychologists on the correct way to carry out treatment and there have been few, if any, really well controlled studies of the beneficial effect of therapy.

At the basic level, the simple understanding by the family that emotional factors may be aggravating the child's asthma can do a lot to help. Parents are often aware of this already and may go out of their way to avoid frustrating or angering the child, but they are then worried about whether or not this is the right thing to do. The sympathetic doctor will listen to the problem and try to help the family take a sensible line. It is best if the parents are brought to realize the best course themselves rather than have it handed to them by the doctor, and this form

The Treatment of the Asthmatic Child

of simple psychotherapy is usually very helpful.

The fact that a high proportion of asthmatic children are very suggestible can be used in the type of treatment known as behaviour therapy. In this technique the patient is taught to relax while he imagines himself in situations which he believes will cause him to wheeze. Over a few weeks, he gradually builds up an imaginary resistance to developing attacks which may then protect him from real attacks. This type of treatment can sometimes enable the doctor to achieve much better control of the asthma with less need for drugs even if it does not completely prevent attacks. Of course, the most attractive method of treating suggestible patients is to hypnotize them and tell them that they will no longer wheeze. There is no doubt that hypnosis can stop or prevent attacks in some patients, but only a few people are sufficiently suggestible to benefit from this treatment, and it is difficult to use in children. If hypnosis is to be tried it must be carried out by a fully qualified doctor who understands both the emotional and physical problems of the patient.

There is little to recommend the more exotic forms of psychotherapy such as Freudian analysis for the treatment of childhood asthma. Most theories on which such treatment is based are not founded on scientific facts as far as asthma is concerned. The treatment is very time consuming and expensive, and the results are poor for all but a few patients.

Various physical forms of treatment such as breathing exercises or athletic training are sometimes recommended for asthmatic children. There is something particularly appealing about breathing exercises for a disease in which the child finds it difficult to breathe and many children have spent many hours learning to regulate their respiration. Unfortunately, breathing exercises are as much part of the folklore of asthma as drugs like the antihistamines, in the sense that they have a small part to play but not nearly as much as some people believe. The

Your Child With Asthma

problem in asthma is due to narrowing of the bronchial tubes and no amount of controlled breathing can make any difference to this fact. However, as was pointed out in Chapter 1, if excessive force is used to try to overcome the obstruction when breathing out it may actually make things worse by compressing the bronchial tubes even further. It is for this reason that a slow, steady expiration is better than the breathing sometimes adopted by the anxious patient during an attack, and trained physiotherapists can help children to breathe more economically. The breathing exercises will do nothing to cure the asthma or prevent attacks recurring and will not develop the child's lungs as some parents believe. When used with all the other effective types of treatment described in this chapter, they may provide some additional help.

Physiotherapy for the lungs is also used during attacks of asthma which are accompanied by a lot of secretions in the lungs or if the child also has a chest infection. The physiotherapist can help to remove secretions by positioning the child and percussing the chest. She is also often the best person to help the child inhale bronchodilator drugs being used for the treatment of an acute attack. These types of physiotherapy are usually carried out in hospital and may be an essential part of the management of the difficult patient.

Some parents and teachers believe that the asthmatic child is basically a weakling and that all his troubles would end if he could be made tougher. This is very far from the truth because the asthmatic's inability to take part in sports and strenuous activities is not due to lack of willing but to the fact that exercise is a very potent stimulus for causing acute asthma. Every effort should be made by doctors to ensure that the child can lead a normal life and take part in physical activities with the help of drugs if necessary, but this may be impossible to achieve completely. No asthmatic child should be compelled to take part in an activity which causes him to become wheezy because the reactions can sometimes be very severe. On the other hand, there is no reason why he should not do things which do not cause attacks and asthmatics often find that swimming is a particularly good sport for them.

The importance of the emotional factor should never be forgotten by people who claim success for the various kinds of treatment such as breathing exercises, physical training or unproven drugs. Parents should beware of claims of this kind and should always consult their doctor about the true place of any treatment being considered.

The Treatment of Status Asthmaticus

Sometimes the asthmatic child develops a really severe attack which requires hospital treatment and if this attack does not respond to simple drugs any longer it is usually called status asthmaticus. Often this develops out of what seems to be an ordinary attack, but occasionally it may be very severe right from the start. Because the treatment is rather different from that normally used for the child at home, it is worthwhile considering it separately.

When the child is brought to hospital in a severe attack, he is usually given an injection of adrenaline (epinephrine) first of all to see if he is still responsive to this type of drug. If not, he may then be given an injection of aminophylline because this sometimes works, but doctors are generally wary of giving much of this drug by injection. Once the decision is made that the child really does have status asthmaticus and is not going to recover rapidly with simple treatment, then he will usually be admitted to the children's ward and treated with steroids. Because of the need for rapid action, the initial dose is often given by injection and if the child has not been drinking much it is usual to give him a constant drip of fluid into a vein and to put his drugs into this fluid. If he is very distressed and not getting enough oxygen, he will be treated in an oxygen tent and he may also be given physiotherapy. Various blood tests and X-rays will be carried out and his treatment will be adjusted according to the results. As soon as he begins to improve, the intensity of treatment is reduced. The infusion into the vein is removed, he is given his drugs by mouth, and he is taken out of the oxygen tent. The high dose of steroid which he was given at first is rapidly reduced and may be stopped completely if he does not need it regularly. He will be allowed home when he is sufficiently improved with a recommendation for his future treatment. When this approach to status asthmaticus is taken it is very unusual for any more intensive treatment to be needed, but in rare cases of extremely severe attacks it is sometimes necessary for the child to be given artificial respiration by a machine if he cannot breathe enough on his own.

This brief account of very severe asthma has been included to give parents some idea of what to expect should this happen to their child, but it must be emphasized that it only occurs in a very small number of children. The vast majority are perfectly well controlled on one or other of the regular treatments discussed earlier in this chapter until they eventually grow out of their asthma.

The Treatment of Eczema and Hay Fever

Although this book is primarily concerned with the problems of asthma, the associated skin condition of eczema, and watering eyes and nose due to hay fever, which commonly occur in asthmatic children, can sometimes give so much trouble that a few comments on their treatment have been included. The type of eczema which occurs in association with asthma in children usually appears at a very young age, and disappears again rather earlier than the asthma itself, but unfortunately it can be quite resistant to treatment. If it is only

The Treatment of the Asthmatic Child

mild, then it may not require any treatment, but when it is widespread or causes severe irritation or is very unsightly then something must be done. The usual approach is to try creams or ointments containing one or other of the steroid drugs, which have been found to be particularly helpful for eczema. There is generally some individual variation in response and it may be necessary to try several different preparations before the best one is found for the individual child. The cream generally needs to be applied twice a day when the eczema is active, but can be stopped when the condition improves. Sometimes the skin may become quite infected, and advice from the doctor should then be taken about the need for antibiotics. In some very resistant cases of eczema, it may be necessary to use softening ointments and these can effectively be applied by putting them into the bath. Occasionally the only method of clearing up really resistant eczema on the arms and legs is to apply the ointment and then cover the limbs in polythene bandages overnight to allow them to soak into the skin. This type of treatment is not usually very practical at home, but can be very helpful during a short stay in hospital for clearing up the eczema. The use of steroid drugs on the skin does not result in the kind of side effects that can be obtained when they are taken by mouth, provided they are used properly under doctor's instructions. Very occasionally it may be necessary to treat the eczema by steroids taken by mouth, in which case the principal of treatment would be just the same as for asthma, which has been discussed earlier.

Hay-fever is the name given to the watering of the eyes and nose in the springtime due to allergy to pollens, which occurs quite often in association with asthma. Provided the symptoms occur at one particular time of year and the child can be shown to be allergic to a particular pollen or pollens, then there is a very good chance of successful treatment by desensitization injections. These injections are normally carried out over the winter months, before the pollen season, to provide the necessary protection. If the child is not desensitized or not controlled in this way, then it may be necessary to take the antihistamine type of medicine to control the symptoms during the pollen season. These tend to make the child drowsy, and should not be continued longer than necessary. They do not have any effect on the asthma itself.

CHAPTER 6

Who Should Treat the Asthmatic Child—and Where?

In the previous chapter it was pointed out that there are a number of different ways in which the asthmatic child may be treated, depending upon the nature of his case, and this also means that a number of different people may be involved in the treatment. This chapter is designed to give parents some idea of the roles of the various people who may treat their child, and the various places in which treatment may be carried out.

The Parent's Role

The most important people by far in the management of the asthmatic child are, of course, his parents. They see much more of him than anyone else and they have to deal with all the day to day problems that arise. The child looks to his parents for help when he is ill and he expects them to know exactly what to do to help him. Children hate to be separated from their parents and would prefer to be very wheezy at home rather than to go into hospital for treatment. All these factors place a very heavy responsibility on the shoulders of the parents, particularly the mother to whom the child generally turns.

The essential job of parents is to ensure that their child is getting the best possible treatment, and in the more troublesome types of asthma it will mean paying attention to many aspects of the disease discussed in this book. In the

Your Child With Asthma

younger child the parents will have to take full responsibility for ensuring that he takes any drugs that he needs and they will have to take note of how effective they are. Older children often become very expert in managing their own illness and parents will just need to keep a general eye on them to make sure that all is well.

Parents must know what to do to help their child if he gets an attack and they must understand the use of any drugs with which he is being treated. They should also know the names and doses of all the drugs in case they have to consult a strange doctor who is not familiar with the case. It is important for the parents to know the pattern of their child's asthma so that they know what to expect and when to start treatment or increase the dose of any drugs which he is taking regularly. If the child can see that his parents know how to deal with his problems, he will have confidence in them and this will remove much of the anxiety which can make attacks so much worse. It is also vital that parents know when things are getting too difficult for them to handle so that they consult their doctor in good time. This often takes some time to learn and in the beginning it is better if they consult their doctor too often rather than allow their child to become severely ill by being over-confident. Later on, most parents acquire an instinct for knowing when to call for help. No hard and fast rules can be given but, in general, if the child is getting worse over the course of a day despite adequate doses of the drugs which have been prescribed for attacks, then the doctor should be consulted.

The role of the parents also includes attention to their child's general social and emotional development. They must realize that they have a child with a handicap which is quite mild in most cases and which he is very likely to grow out of as time goes by. They must not allow his schooling or play to be neglected because he is supposed to be a "delicate" child and they may have to take extra trouble to help him keep up with his friends. Some parents are too over-protective towards their children and make them too babyish and dependent, while others are too harsh and unsympathetic and may make them unhappy and nervous. The majority of parents treat their children with common sense so that the child knows he can trust them and they know when the child really needs attention. In this type of family there is every chance of the child ending up as a perfectly healthy teenager without any physical or emotional handicaps.

The Family Doctor's Role

In the United Kingdom most asthmatic children are under the direct supervision of their family general practitioner. In other countries such as the U.S.A. they will be under the care of a family doctor with a special interest in children. The roles of these different types of family doctor are essentially the same, that is to provide the main part of the child's management on the basis of a very good knowledge of both him and his family. After all, it is usually the general practitioner who is called out in the middle of the night when the child is ill and who knows what the home circumstances are like, not the hospital doctors.

Most general practitioners have a fair amount of experience in handling asthmatic children because it is the commonest of all long-term problems in this age group. They usually have a pretty good idea of how bad the condition is and what factors such as infection, allergy, or emotion, are important in the individual case. When the general practitioner feels that more detailed investigation is required, he will usually recommend a hospital consultation and will act on the information which is passed to him. Because it is the family doctor to whom parents turn for advice it is essential that there is very good communication between him and the hospital doctors so that each knows what the other thinks about the child. In some cases the school doctors are also following the child's progress and they too will keep in touch with the general practitioner. It can be seen that he acts as the one person to whom all information should be channelled so that he is in the best position to give the family the correct advice.

When the general practitioner is called in because the child is wheezy, he must decide whether or not treatment should be carried out at home or in hospital. It is essential that he sees the child in good time if he is to start effective home treatment. The decision about admission to hospital will be based on his knowledge of the child's likely response to treatment and the facilities available at home.

Some parents expect their family doctor to know all about every disease and cannot see why it is necessary for him to refer the child to hospital. Medical care is a very large subject which is changing almost daily and it is quite impossible for any doctor to keep completely up to date on all aspects. The wise general practitioner will know enough about new developments so that he can decide when there is a chance that his patient will benefit from a consultation with a specialist in the subject. Because of the nature of asthma it is often useful for the child to continue to attend the specialist clinic for observation, but the good specialist will make these visits as far apart as possible and rely on the family doctor to take primary care of the child.

The Specialist's Role

From discussions in earlier chapters it can be seen that asthma is a disease which may involve different kinds of specialists, such as doctors dealing with allergy, chest illnesses or breathing tests. Where children are concerned, most doctors believe that they should be seen by a specialist in children's diseases because it is important to understand the whole patient.

Who Should Treat the Asthmatic Child—and Where?

This immediately raises problems because the children's specialist (paediatrician) has to take care of all kinds of problems and so his knowledge about asthma may not be as detailed as that of the adult's doctor who has specialized in chest diseases. Because asthma is such an important disease in childhood, many paediatricians are very interested in the subject and may well run special clinics for asthmatic children in which they have the ability to carry out any tests that are needed. Alternatively, they may work together with adult's specialists who can provide extra help.

Because so many parents and doctors have been led to believe that asthma is all due to allergy, it is quite common for children to be referred to an allergist for investigation. These doctors are usually very skilled in sorting out the real place of allergy in the individual and in deciding on the value of desensitization or other types of treatment. With the great advances that have been made in drug treatment of asthma, many allergists use drugs in addition to allergic management, and the difference between the allergist and the specialist in chest diseases is becoming much less obvious.

The role of the hospital specialist as far as routine outpatient consultations are concerned is really to decide on the severity of the condition and to recommend treatment. He will gather as much information as he can from his interview with the family and from the various tests which are carried out, and with the help of the opinion of the general practitioner he will try to give the correct advice. In some cases this will involve starting on a course of a long-term treatment which may need regular visits to the hospital for supervision, but the specialist should encourage the major part of treatment to be give by the family doctor. In cases where the child is admitted to hospital with severe asthma, it is usually the hospital specialist who takes charge and decides on which of the various forms of treatment are needed. Before discharging the child he should also be sure that adequate arrangements have been made for future supervision by the family doctor and the hospital clinic if necessary. The hospital doctor has a special responsibility to see that the child is well in other ways apart from his asthma and this is why it is generally a good idea for the specialist to be an expert in children's diseases.

Besides hospital specialists dealing with the asthma itself there are a number of other experts who may need to be consulted. The importance of emotional factors in asthma means that it is generally worthwhile investigating this aspect of the problem. Because of the skill required to do this properly, it is usually carried out by a clinical psychologist. By means of standard tests and interviews, the psychologist attempts to define the importance of emotional factors and usually also looks into the question of school performance at the same time. The findings are reported to the specialist in charge of the child and if treatment is required then the psychologist will often carry it out. In some cases the child may also be seen by a child psychiatrist who is a doctor specializing in emotional problems in children. The psychiatrist, the psychologist and the social worker usually co-operate very closely with each other and with the school medical services.

When an asthmatic child also has severe eczema it may be necessary for him to be seen by a skin specialist. Treatment is usually carried out on an out-patient basis, but occasionally the problem is so bad that the only thing to do is to admit the child to hospital. Other specialists may also become involved because the asthmatic child is just as likely as any other to develop illnesses which are not associated with asthma. A common problem that arises is the need for dental treatment, especially when this involves an anaesthetic to have teeth out. This rarely causes any trouble but it is often a good idea if it is carried out in hospital, especially if the child is being treated with steroid drugs.

Who Should Treat the Asthmatic Child—and Where?

The School's Role

Asthma is such a common condition in childhood that every school can expect about 5 to 10 out of every 100 children to have the disease and about 1 in every 100 to have it badly enough to need treatment from time to time. This means that teachers must have some idea about the nature of asthma and the kind of problem that may arise with their pupils. They are in a very similar position to parents in this respect. Teachers have a special responsibility because they have to decide if a child is fit enough to stay at school or whether they should contact the parents to take him home. Parents are sometimes upset because they believe the teacher is making too much or too little fuss about their child, but the decision is difficult for someone without medical training and teachers have to learn by experience.

It is essential that the school appreciates the problems of the asthmatic child and helps him to lead as normal a life as possible. Young children are very unsympathetic towards each other and the teacher may have to protect the asthmatic from being teased or bullied. The severity of exercise provoked asthma also means that the child may not be able to keep up with sports and games and should not be forced to do so if it is known that this makes him wheeze. On the other hand, he should be encouraged in those activities at which he can compete and taught to stand up for himself as much as possible. It may be necessary for the child to take drugs at school and it is often best if these are kept by the class teacher or by the school nurse if there is one available. In this way there is less likelihood that doses will be forgotten or lost. Parents are sometimes unwilling to let their children take medicines to school because they think it will be "too much trouble", but this is quite wrong, especially for preventative drugs like Intal or for steroids which often have to be taken at regular intervals throughout the day if they are to work properly.

Most schools arrange for regular medical examinations to be carried out on their children and the school medical service does very valuable work in bringing some unrecognized problems to the attention of family doctors and hospital specialists. They are in a very good position to judge the effect of ill health on the child's school work and may sometimes advise special schooling if they feel he is unable to cope because of frequent absences.

Where Should the Asthmatic Child be Treated?

Just as there are a number of different ways of treating asthma and a number of people who may be involved in the treatment, so there are also a number of different places where treatment can be carried out. It goes almost without saying that the best place for a child is in his own home and the most satisfactory type of treatment is one which allows him to live at home and attend his normal school. In some cases it may be necessary for the child to be treated elsewhere and parents need to understand why this may be required.

From what has been discussed earlier, it is clear that the large majority of asthmatic children have the disease in a mild form and are managed very satisfactorily by their parents and their family doctor. Once the diagnosis has been made and the best form of treatment has been found, the child can live a normal life apart from occasional visits to the doctor's surgery (office) for a check-up or to renew his medicines. It is a good idea if the parents know the usual treatment that their child needs so that they can explain it to a strange doctor that they may need to consult when away from home or when their own doctor is not available. If this type of mild asthmatic child has a more serious attack, then it will usually be possible for him to be treated at home by the family doctor who will keep an eye on

Who Should Treat the Asthmatic Child—and Where?

him until he is sure the attack is passing over. Even if the child needs an injection, this will often be given by the family doctor at home or in his surgery and, provided the attack improves quickly, there is no reason why he should need to go to hospital.

From time to time an asthmatic child may have quite a severe attack and will need to attend the hospital Emergency Department, either because his own doctor feels that more intensive treatment may be needed or because his own doctor cannot be contacted in time. It is difficult for parents to know how long they should delay going to hospital if they cannot contact their own doctor for some reason. A reasonable suggestion would be to take the child to the hospital if he is having an attack which is more severe than usual and getting worse despite using his regular treatment and if it is unlikely that the family doctor would be able to see the child for about 2 or 3 hours. It is impossible to make hard and fast rules about this but most "asthmatic" parents soon come to know when the situation is becoming urgent. Emergency Department treatment is not a particularly satisfactory method of dealing with the asthmatic child because the doctors there often know nothing of his previous illness and treatment, and the whole atmosphere of these departments is rather frightening for children. They come to associate hospital with doctors in white coats who give injections and this may make it difficult if the child needs to attend again. When the child is seen in the Emergency Department, the doctors will decide on what treatment is needed and, provided the child responds quickly, he will usually be allowed to go home. If the attack is more severe, they will usually decide that the child should be admitted to the children's ward. Even if the child is allowed home, the Emergency Department doctor will want to know that the child has really recovered and he will often arrange for a follow-up visit to the children's out-patient clinic or the asthma clinic.

Your Child With Asthma

The asthma clinic is used to assess the severity of the asthma and decide on treatment in new patients referred by their family doctor, and to follow the progress of the child until it is clear that all is going well. Parents often come to rely very heavily on the doctor in the asthma clinic and it is important that they should have very free access to him. They should not be kept waiting for weeks for an appointment and they should be able to arrange to attend earlier than the date fixed if they are worried. It is also helpful if they can telephone for advice if necessary, even though that advice will almost always be to go and see their own family doctor first. When the asthma clinic is arranged along these lines, there is a temptation for the clinic doctor to replace the family doctor in some ways, but this is quite wrong because the family doctor will almost always be the first line of defence in a crisis. This means that there must be very good communication between the clinic and family doctor so that they can jointly provide all the help that parents may need.

If the child is having a bad attack, he will often need to be admitted to the hospital. With very few exceptions he will be best off in the children's ward along with other children where the nurses and doctors are familiar with handling sick and unhappy children. Most children's wards now have a very liberal policy about visiting and there is no doubt that it is best if one or both parents spend as much time as possible with their child. Of course they may have to leave the bedside when essential nursing or medical procedures are being carried out and there is little point in staying at night once the child has fallen asleep. It is very important that parents avoid misleading their child about what is going to happen and that they explain everything in simple and reassuring terms. They should not use the threat of admission to hospital to scare the child if he misbehaves at home and equally they should not tell him that he won't have any injections in the ward when the doctor has told them that this will be necessary. The child must be able to rely on his parents and have confidence in them and then admission to the children's ward will not be too unpleasant. As soon as he has made a satisfactory recovery, he will be allowed to go home but it is important that this is not rushed because it is sometimes necessary to readmit the child if he has been discharged too early. After leaving the hospital, he will usually be given a follow-up appointment for the asthma clinic to make sure that he remains well.

Special Schools, Boarding Schools and Sanatoria

The question is frequently raised about whether or not an asthmatic child should be sent to a special school. In the large majority of cases there is no need for this because the child can attend his ordinary school, and the less disturbance made in his everyday life the better. It is only when the asthma is so bad or so frequent that the child cannot keep up with normal schooling that the question of a special school has to be given serious consideration. Even then, because of the benefits of normal schooling, every effort must be made to improve the child's treatment so that he can cope with his ordinary school, before recommending a special school. The advantage of a special school for the severely affected child is that the staff are trained to cope with the medical and educational problems that can arise and this may mean that he receives a better education. The fact that such day schools are often called "open-air" schools or schools for "delicate" children really has nothing whatever to do with the management of asthmatic children. There is not a shred of scientific evidence that "open-air" ever did any asthmatic child any good, and it may even induce an attack in a child who is particularly sensitive to changes of air temperature. The belief in "open-air" largely stems from the days when there was no effective treatment for asthma in the form of modern drugs. It is the skill of the staff of these special schools, not the "air", which makes all the difference for the few very severely affected asthmatics. Special schools should not be used as a method of getting rid of difficult children from ordinary schools just because the staff find it a bit inconvenient. Even the best of the special schools places the child at some disadvantage because of all the other sick children there who may not be able to maintain a normal pace of education in class.

Another type of special school which may be of use in the occasional child is the residential boarding school. For reasons which have never been satisfactorily explained, some children do much better away from home even when there are no obvious emotional factors or allergic factors involved. This is clearly a drastic step for most families to take and residential schooling should only be arranged when all other reasonable alternatives have been explored. It should probably be reserved for those few children who cannot be controlled at home without the use of such large doses of steroid drugs that they are at risk of developing serious side effects. This condition is becoming even more rare now with the newer and safer drugs that are being produced. In these few children the move to a residential school can have an almost miraculous effect and in many cases they are able to make large reductions or even stop their drugs. A particular problem in this situation is that the child often gets very bad again if he returns home during the school holidays and parents have to be prepared to restart all his old treatment immediately, even on the way home in the train. Some residential schools are associated with hospitals and there are some long-term hospitals for children which serve much the same function but arrange for their patients to attend the local school. Children should not spend long periods in an ordinary hospital because the facilities for education and recreation are never as good as those at regular schools or

Who Should Treat the Asthmatic Child—and Where?

special schools. In the United Kingdom, quite a number of healthy children are sent to private boarding schools and this sometimes deals very effectively with the problem of the asthmatic child of the more well-off parents. In general, parents should not send their asthmatic child to such a school unless he would normally be going there, because if the child is really in need of special residential schooling it is best (and usually free) if this is arranged through the school medical services.

Finally, there are a number of fashionable resorts in Europe and America which are supposed to be good for asthmatic children. When tuberculosis stopped being a problem because of the discovery of effective drugs, many of the old tuberculosis sanatoria in Switzerland and similar places were converted to treat asthmatic children. It must be clearly understood that there is nothing magic in these institutions and equal success with treatment could be obtained by sending the children away from home to almost anywhere. Much of the apparent success of foreign resorts is due to removing the child from home and the remainder of any success is probably due to the fact that most children grow out of their asthma over a period of time. With few exceptions, it is wrong to send a child far away from home to receive treatment that he could almost certainly get just as well while living with his family, or, in very severe cases, from a special or residential school within easy reach of his family.

CHAPTER 7

Some Important Rules for Parents

Reading through the previous chapters of this book, the parent of the asthmatic child will realize that there are still a few mysteries about asthma but, on the whole, we now know a great deal about it. In the past when we were more ignorant there was a tendency to develop vague ideas about the causes of asthma and to propose various forms of treatment which had no scientific value. Nowadays our whole approach is based on an understanding of the bodily mechanisms which cause the wheezing and the way in which drugs or other forms of treatment can relieve it.

It is unreasonable to expect parents to grasp the whole of the contents of this book and to plan their handling of their asthmatic child in the various ways which have been discussed. There are, however, a few very important basic ideas which it is well worth emphasizing again, and so the following set of "rules" has been put together as the parting message.

(1) KNOW YOUR DOCTOR:

Parents should know the name and telephone number of their regular family doctor and where he can be contacted in an emergency. They should also know how to contact his deputy if he is away, and they should take steps to find out where they could contact a doctor who would understand the problem if their child should need attention while away from home, for

Some Important Rules for Parents

example when on holiday. In almost all circumstances it is best to contact the family doctor first, but parents should also know the name and telephone number of the doctor they regularly see in the asthma clinic.

(2) KNOW YOUR DRUGS:

It is extremely helpful and may even be vital for parents to know the names and doses of any drugs that their child is receiving. They should ask the doctor who prescribes them to write down the real medical name for the drug and not just a trade name or some general term such as "antibiotics". Since tablets and medicines often come in different strengths, parents should also be sure that they know the quantity of drug in each pill or mixture. It is important to know how often the drug should be taken and whether or not it is permitted to increase the number of doses taken in a day.

(3) MAINTAIN YOUR STOCK:

When the child needs drugs to treat his asthma, it is important that an adequate supply is kept at home, even if they are only needed very occasionally. Running out of drugs is often just inconvenient, but could be very dangerous in some situations. Attacks of asthma can occur at any time and it may be difficult to renew supplies during the night or at weekends. If the child is on regular daily treatment with drugs, don't wait until you have run out before getting a new supply.

(4) GIVE DETAILS OF TREATMENT TO ANY STRANGE DOCTOR CONSULTED:

Should the child need medical attention from a doctor who is not familiar with his case, it is vital that parents are able to tell this doctor as much as possible about their child's treatment. This is especially important if the child has to be seen because of something unrelated to asthma, for example if he has an accident or needs to have an operation. If the child is being treated with the steroid drugs or has taken them regularly in the previous year, it is essential to let any new doctor know about it, particularly if the child is going to need an anaesthetic. This also applies to a dental operation if the child is going to be asleep for the treatment.

(5) DON'T STOP TREATMENT SUDDENLY:

Unless you are told otherwise by your usual doctor, it is unwise to stop any drug suddenly. This is particularly important for the preventative drug Intal and for most types of steroid drugs because the asthma attack may return very rapidly. It is quite safe to stop these drugs over a period of a few days on doctor's advice and it may also be safe to stop steroids suddenly if they have only been taken for a short time. This is a medical decision, however, and parents should rely on expert advice.

(6) KNOW WHAT TO DO FOR AN ATTACK:

Even if the child's asthma is well under control parents should ask their doctor what to do if he gets worse or develops a severe attack. Usually this will mean increasing his regular drugs and parents should be sure how to do this safely and effectively. In some cases it will mean adding stand-by drugs to his usual treatment for a few days. Every attempt should be made to keep the child taking Intal or steroids during an attack if he was on them before. If this is difficult because of severe wheeze or vomiting, the doctor should be consulted at once. It is generally safe to increase the number of doses of selective

Some Important Rules for Parents

bronchodilator drugs such as salbutamol but there are risks with the older drugs like isoprenaline (isoproterenol). The size and frequency of the dose recommended by your doctor for dealing with an attack should not be exceeded.

(7) KNOW WHEN TO CALL THE DOCTOR:

There is no doubt that some of the most difficult attacks occur in the children of the most capable parents because they tend to continue to treat their child for too long before calling the doctor. If the child is not improving over a few hours despite the recommended treatment, it is usually worth speaking to the doctor about it. This is more important in the evening or before the weekend when it may be difficult to contact him if things get really bad.

(8) DON'T TAKE ADVICE FROM AMATEURS:

There are a great many old wive's tales about asthma which are at best useless and at worst dangerous. It is very unwise for parents to seek or take advice from anyone other than a medically qualified doctor. This applies particularly to anyone offering to "cure" the child by means of patent medicines, faith healing or hypnotism. There is no "cure" for asthma, only treatment to relieve it until the child grows out of it, and hypnotism can be very dangerous unless carried out by a doctor with special training. Parents often waste a lot of money buying patent medicines or substances to rub on the chest which are supposed to help the "chesty" child. The regulations controlling the sale of drugs are very strict and anything which can be bought without a doctor's prescription must be so bland that it cannot contain enough of any of the drugs which are really effective in asthma. If your child needs drugs, get them from your doctor.

(9) REMEMBER: YOUR CHILD PROBABLY HAS 9 OUT OF 10 CHANCES OR BETTER OF COMPLETELY LOSING HIS ASTHMA BY THE TIME HE REACHES HIS TEENS.

INDEX

Allergy in asthma, 10–3
    tests, 38
    treatment, 51
Alveolus (air sac), 2
Antibiotics, 60
Antihistamines, 61
Asthma clinic, 32–4

Blood tests, 37
Breathing exercises, 63
Bronchial constriction, 5–6
    dilatation, 7
Bronchodilator drugs, 54
Bronchus (airway), 2

Causes of asthma, 9–21
Chest infection, 13–4

Deaths from asthma, 31
Desensitization for allergy, 52
Diary card, 34
Drugs for asthma, 53–62

Emotional factors in asthma, 14–6
Environmental factors in asthma, 17–9

Eczema, 24
    treatment, 66
Exercise factors in asthma, 8, 18–9
    tests, 45

Hay fever treatment, 67
House-dust allergy, 12

Infection in asthma, 13
Inherited factors in asthma, 19
Intal (sodium cromoglycate), 56
Investigation of asthma, 32–48

Lung function in asthma, 6–8
    in health, 2–5
    tests, 42

Medical history questions, 32–3

Oxygen and Carbon Dioxide exchange, 4

Patterns of asthma, 22–31
Peak expiratory flow rate measurement, 43
Peak flow meter, 43
Physical examination, 33–4

Index

Physiotherapy, 64
Psychological tests, 46
   treatment, 62

Rules for parents, 82–6

Schooling for asthmatic children, 79–81

Skin tests for allergy, 11, 38
Status asthmaticus (severe attack), 30

Steroid drugs, 57–60
Structure of lungs in asthma, 6–8
   in health, 2–5

Treatment of asthma, 49–68
   status asthmaticus, 65

Wheezy babies, 22

X-rays, 37